ZOO VET

ZOO VET

Adventures of a
Wild Animal Doctor

DAVID TAYLOR

J. B. Lippincott Company
Philadelphia and New York

U.S. Library of Congress Cataloging in Publication Data

Taylor, David, birth date
    Zoo vet : Adventures of a wild animal doctor.

    1. Zoo animals—Diseases. 2. Taylor, David, birth date
3. Veterinarians—Biography. I. Title.
SF996.T39   1977   636.089′092′4   [B]   76–56834
ISBN–0–397–01207–1

To
H. E. L.

Contents

ZOO
VET

1 A Quarter of a Million Gallons of Blood

"IT'S ALL BLOOD! All the water's turned to blood!" the whale trainer gasped to me over the telephone one morning before breakfast. As a freelance zoo veterinarian flitting about the country from crisis to emergency to disaster daily, I was accustomed to frantic phone calls early in the morning, but this one was new to me. When the trainer had calmed down a little, he said he had walked into the dolphinarium at Flamingo Park Zoo that morning and had had a terrible shock. The deep hourglass-shaped pool in which the killer whale, Cuddles, had lived for three years was no longer brimming with clear-blue artificial sea water. Instead the entire pool was filled with murky scarlet liquid. Something terrible must have happened to the whale; the trainer had expected to find the sixteen-foot-long animal lying disembowelled on the bottom of the pool. But no. With the usual blast of steaming breath, Cuddles' shining black head suddenly emerged from the red soup. He was alive! The trainer had dashed down to the basement and peered anxiously through the underwater windows. It was like looking into a crimson fog, a pea-souper with less than six inches' visibility.

He called me right away, and I set off for the zoo

immediately. Obviously, I thought, someone is exaggerating in the heat of the moment. Whales bleed like any other animal when injured, but to turn 250,000 gallons completely red? Impossible! Nevertheless, I kept my foot hard down on the accelerator as I drove the hundred miles over the Pennine Hills between my home and the zoo, a beautiful park set beneath the North Yorkshire moors. Sheer horror erased all question of exaggeration the instant I saw the pool. It was actually true. The water looked like somewhat thin blood.

Cuddles floated quietly in the middle of the pool. His deep black body colour had taken on more of a dark grey shade and he seemed to be lightening in colour even as one watched. When I called him over to the side he responded sluggishly. This was not the perky, mischievous creature that I knew so well who would call to me with his high-pitched piggy squeal and fix me with one dark and shiny eye whenever I passed through the crowd of spectators. He was torpid and depressed. His gums and the membrane round his eye, normally a deep pink colour, were now a deathly white. I inquired about his appetite. Zero. For the first time since he had arrived in Yorkshire, Cuddles' enormous appetite for herring and mackerel had vanished. Normally a glutton who could clear eighty pounds of fish at a go, now he could not face even a single fish.

I was alarmed. Of all the animals with which I had worked, I had been closest to Cuddles. Despite the species' fearsome-sounding name, and although in the wild state they are voracious and deadly hunters, killer whales in captivity are generally amenable and gentle towards the humans who look after them. I had been with Cuddles when he arrived one frosty winter night, a plump and genial baby with teeth just cutting through his gums. During the summers we had played together in the water every day. He loved to hug me with his flippers while he floated vertically and I tickled his smooth round belly with my toes. He also enjoyed carrying a rider on his back, either in front of his dorsal fin or behind on what I called the rumble seat, where the ride was bumpy and exhilarating.

As a patient he had been impeccable. We had designed a special examination sling that ran out over Cuddles' pool on telescopic girders. Not only was he easy to get into this device for routine blood sampling or vaccination, or for the removal of minor warts, but he was positively reluctant to leave this aquatic examination couch. We had always had to entice him out of, rather than into, it. I had learned most of my techniques of whale handling and medication on Cuddles, overhauling him from tip to toe every month, dressing every scratch or pimple that he developed, no matter how minute, rooting out every last worm or fluke that tried to parasitize him. I had set up a rigorous food-inspection system which ensured him fish of a quality higher than that enjoyed by diners at the finest London restaurants, and guaranteed to be free from hidden mackerel hooks and other stray bits of metal fishing tackle which might, if swallowed, pose a deadly threat to the animal's intestines. I'd had headaches and heartaches and missed meals and sleepless nights over this animal, with his occasional sore eye or chipped tooth or bout of diarrhoea. He'd been pampered and cosseted and watched over, and now it seemed that I was about to lose him through some mysterious calamity.

The first priority was to find out where the blood was coming from. There was no sign of a wound on his upper surface as he bobbed slowly in the water. I put on a wet suit and jumped into the pool. The crimson water smelt sour and unpleasant. I paddled across to my friend and hugged his head. Cuddles gazed at me with his round dark eyes but made no move to snuggle up to me as he usually did. Ominously, the healthy syrupy tears no longer flowed from his eyelids. Cuddles was dehydrating somehow, bleeding to death.

I went all over his back and tail flukes: no sign of any injury. Then, using his paddle-like left flipper as a lever, I laboriously rolled him over in the water. His gleaming white abdomen broke the water surface. Not a trace of a wound could I see. There were now only two possibilities: The blood was coming out either with his urine or in his stools. Suddenly, as he floated like a great capsized plastic boat, a massive welter of what seemed to be pure blood gushed out of his anus. That was it. Cuddles was bleeding massively somewhere in his intestines.

Climbing out of the pool, I gave instructions for it to be emptied immediately. While the water was going down I filled a syringe with a potent dose of a chemical that increases the clotting speed of blood, and using my dart-gun I shot it into the back muscles of the whale as he surfaced. Whatever the problem was, it had struck rapidly out of the blue. Cuddles had been normal up to the previous evening when the dolphinarium staff went home. It seemed to be affecting the lower bowel; if the bleeding source was in the stomach or high in the bowel the blood would have been partly digested and changed to a much darker brown or black colour on its way through the intestinal tract. I suspected a bacterial or virus infection producing rapid ulceration of the bowel lining. If it was a bacterium, perhaps the culprit was the evil Salmonella, a food-poisoning germ which causes diarrhoea and the passing of blood in other animals.

Whatever the cause, my first priority now was to get Cuddles down onto the dry bottom of the pool, examine him thoroughly, and take blood samples to see how bad the damage was; in his apathetic state there was no chance of luring him into the telescopic sling. Next I had to stop the bleeding and replace some of the liquid that his circulation had lost. When the volume of circulating blood becomes too small to carry enough oxygen and other vital supplies to key organs, shock and death speedily set in. How to expand Cuddles' blood volume? I decided that I had to make preparations for some sort of transfusion, but killer whale blood is not quite the sort of stuff that is usually available at the local blood bank. The nearest captive killers were in America. Perhaps one of my colleagues out there had some suitable blood stored.

I telephoned all the major marinelands in the United States and explained my predicament. No one had any killer whale blood stored and no one had come across a similar problem. My friend Dr. White at the Miami Seaquarium had had a case of severe bleeding in a whale that had crashed through an underwater viewing window. It had needed lots of surgery and supportive medical therapy, but no blood transfusions had been given. Would anyone fancy volunteering one of their whales as the donor of one or two dozen pints? I could easily get the stuff shipped over express on the next Pan-Am or TWA flight. The answer was always the same. Highly valuable animals. The difficulty of having to drain pools in the middle of the show season in order to take blood. Anyway, how were we to know, without wasting days testing samples, whether any particular whale's blood would be compatible with Cuddles'? We knew that there were certainly three major blood groups in bottle-nosed dolphins, but no one knew anything about the blood groups of whales. Whole blood transfusion was out.

The fire brigade arrived. Whenever we needed to speed up the emptying of the pools they were called in. Half an hour later, an unusually pale whale lay passively on the concrete bottom of the pool while hoses and buckets were used to keep his skin moist. I went down and took blood from the big blood vessel in his tail. Even to the naked eye the sample appeared watery and thin. The crucial analyses were quickly done in the laboratory at the pool side. As I had feared, Cuddles had lost a great deal of blood into the intestines. Normally he carried seventeen grammes of hae-moglobin, the red oxygen-carrying constituent, in every hundred cc's of his blood. Now it was down to only ten grammes. The total number of red blood cells had also dropped precipitously. Other tests showed no sign of ac-tive bacterial infection or liver or kidney damage.

A trainer came into the laboratory carrying what looked like a fragment of wet white paper. "He's just passed another load of blood," he reported, "and there was this in it."

The specimen was sticky and fragile. I dropped it into a beaker of cold water and teased it out with a needle. It unfolded into a delicate white film as big as a postage stamp. The film was not completely intact for at three or four points there were round holes ringed distinctly by reddish-brown material. It was a piece of intestinal lining mem-brane, and the holes were ulcers surrounded by blood pig-ment, a valuable find but a depressing one. Cuddles had actively bleeding multiple ulcers in his bowels. If there were so many on this small fragment, how many thousands more might there be if the entire hundred feet of his in-testines were similarly involved?

The bit of bowel lining and some swabs went to the bacteriology laboratory for urgent examination and I then returned to the problem of replacing Cuddles' lost blood volume. Since a whole blood transfusion wasn't possible, I had to take second best. Although it had no oxygen-carry-ing power, a transfusion of artificial plasma would combat many of the shock-producing factors and stop the blood vessels from literally collapsing. It was going to mean putting Cuddles on an intravenous drip; at least forty pints would be required. An urgent call for help was sent out to Leeds General Hospital. They readily agreed to supply us with a hundred bottles of the life-saving liquid and it was dispatched by fast car under police escort. Meanwhile I filled Cuddles with other drugs to tackle the sadly abused bowels. Through the giant one-foot-long needle I injected vitamins, anti-inflammatory drugs, and antibiotics. And, although it would take ten to fourteen days to be assembled into the essential haemoglobin, I gave big shots of liquid iron salts. He would need the iron reserves if he recovered.

When the cases of artificial plasma arrived I started work on the transfusion. I used a special needle-like tube of the sort we had employed when doing electrocardiographic investigations on Cuddles some weeks before. The tube had to be inserted accurately into a tail vein. In both dolphins and killer whales, veins and arteries near the surface are closely intermingled for heat-exchange purposes. It is easy to accidentally place a needle into the wrong type of blood vessel, and if any of the liquid from an intravenous injection goes into an artery there can be nasty repercussions, including profound sloughing and death of a large area of tail skin and deeper tissues. With a keeper holding Cuddles' great tail above my head, I knelt and inserted the tube and checked and double-checked to be sure that the blood oozing from it was coming only from a vein. When I was satisfied that all was well I connected the plastic tubes to the plasma bottle and adjusted the dosage regulator. A keeper stood on a chair, holding the bottle high in the air so that the flow of liquid was not counteracted by Cuddles' massive heart pressure.

Slowly the golden fluid seeped into the whale's system. After ten minutes I switched to the second bottle. Although whale blood does not clot easily, I had anticipated trouble with the tube in the vein and had coated it with a chemical to inhibit clotting and consequent blockage. Still, I felt sure that frequent changes of the tube would be necessary.

In fact, as the hours passed slowly by, the keepers holding the bottles and the bottles themselves were the only things that had to be changed. The tube remained unblocked throughout the whole ten hours of the transfusion. Cuddles was as good as gold. Not once did he protest or wriggle.

The man holding the tail up during all this time refused to be relieved. He, too, was deeply involved with the animal and wanted to do everything in his power to help. It was cold and damp in the pool bottom, so I sent for a bottle of rum to ward off inner chills. From time to time I insisted on the tail holder taking a good pull from the rum bottle. So solicitous was I that I did not realize how many tots he had taken during the long hours of waiting. When it was all finished we discovered that the good man was totally drunk and so incapacitated that we had to hoist him out of the pool in a dolphin sling.

We refilled the pool. To my delight, when it was up to the six-foot mark Cuddles accepted a few fish. It was terrible to see the chalk-white back of his throat when he opened his jaws to take them, but at least the boy was eating again. I stopped the refilling at eight feet. It was good to see clear blue water again, but what if he continued to bleed?

I phoned my wife, Shelagh, back at home. I needed to unload my worries on someone. Shelagh has a deep feeling for animals, unlimited resources of common sense, and she had been in on all the past alarums. She had helped revive dying polar bear cubs by dunking them in baths of hot water, had dinner parties and holidays cancelled or curtailed by ungrateful elephants with colic, and had acted as anaesthetist *cum* nurse *cum* cleaner in the middle of the numerous nights when emergency surgery on monkeys or macaws had to be carried out. She'd had young camels crammed into the back of her car and paralysed lion cubs dragging themselves over the kitchen floor, and I'd never heard her complain. We talked over the grim events of the past few hours, and her positive attitude lightened my depression.

"If you feed him by stomach tube," she suggested, "don't forget to add some Guinness like you used to do with the cows."

Not a bad suggestion, I thought. The black Irish beer had been useful in the old days when I had had the problem of reviving weak and debilitated cattle after bad calvings or bleeding milk veins.

Shelagh also informed me that Lindsey, my younger daughter, then eight years old, had arranged for Cuddles to be included in the morning prayers of her class at the convent kindergarten she attended. I still have the card on which Lindsey wrote out the words. The prayer prudently contains a clause requesting that "if Dad doesn't pull it off with the whale and he does die, please let him go to heaven where he belongs." Everything helps when you're up to your neck in it.

The next morning I held my breath as I went into the dolphinarium. My heart sank like an express elevator when I saw the glum expressions on the faces of the trainers. The pool water was deep scarlet again. We drained immediately and once more I took a blood sample. The haemoglobin and red cell counts were lower than before, below the critical point at which, in humans, a blood transfusion becomes imperative. I transfused the plasma again, gave more injections, and inserted a stomach tube. Cuddles took it all placidly. Through the stomach tube I pumped in a peculiar pink mixture which I had concocted in a large unused plastic dustbin. It contained water and honey, mineral salts to replace those lost in the bleeding, glucose, rose-hip syrup, invalid food, kaolin to soothe the inflamed bowel, and Guinness, as Shelagh had suggested. As it by-passed his taste buds I do not suppose Cuddles relished it or otherwise.

The next day things looked much brighter: Cuddles had not bled overnight and showed an improved appetite. The following day dawn broke for the third time on a scene of gory water, but analysis showed the blood loss to have been much reduced and the haemoglobin level, though still below the critical minimum, was levelling out. Still seriously worried, but no longer in complete despair, I repeated my injections and the dustbin mixture.

By now the laboratory results were all back. No bacteria were involved. The cause of the ulcers remained a mystery, as it does to this day, although I strongly believe a virus to have been the culprit. Cuddles continued to eat quite well and even agreed to play gently. He did not haemorrhage on the day after the third bleeding, on the next day, or on the one after that. I became increasingly hopeful. The whale was still very pale but steadily growing stronger, and I fortified his fish by packing them with chunks of cooked Lancashire black puddings, rare delicacies made from blood and fat.

Cuddles never bled again. His recovery was fast and free from further incident. Two weeks after the first attack his blood analysis was halfway back to normal, and in a further three weeks it was completely satisfactory. By this time he was greedily gulping down whole undisguised black puddings by the dozen and opening his now salmon-pink mouth with alacrity to have foaming quarts of Guinness poured straight into his gullet.

There are many things about Cuddles' bleeding disease

I do not understand, and which if any of my lines of treatment helped to save the day will never be known. Certainly the transfusions only averted death from shock and tackled some of the circulatory complications. Perhaps it was the kaolin or the anti-inflammatory drugs or the black puddings that turned the tide against the ulcers. Perhaps if a virus was involved Cuddles developed a rapid immunity which effectively combated the attack.

A Devonshire woman working at Flamingo Park as personal secretary to the director has a different view on the affair. When it was all over, she told me what *she* had done to help the dying killer whale.

"When he bled the third time I went and phoned a wise woman in my home village in the West Country," she said. "She uses white magic on warts and styes and rheumatism. Marvellous reputation. Never known to fail."

"What did you say to her?" I asked.

"I told her briefly what was wrong at the dophinarium and she just said that everything would be all right, and that the bleeding would stop when I put the receiver down."

It sounded like the most ridiculous humbug to me, but I respected the director's secretary as an astute and intelligent woman.

"Well," I said, "can you remember the time when you finished speaking to your wise woman acquaintance?"

"Yes, I can," she replied. "It was eight thirty in the morning."

I walked down to the dolphinarium and looked in the record book. Every minute item concerning the whale and the dolphins in health and sickness is logged there day by day, year in and year out. On the morning of the third and final episode of Cuddles' bleeding a trainer had recorded the last occasion on which the whale was seen to pass blood. The time was entered as 8:31 A.M.

2 Belle Vue Zoo

As a small child I never considered for a moment becoming anything other than a veterinarian—and more than that, I was determined to become a wild animal veterinarian. Close contact with the hair, the warm skin, the chunky muscle of an undomesticated animal gave me a physical thrill—as it does to this day.

I was exceptionally fortunate in that Rochdale, the town in which I was born and grew up, afforded me ample opportunity to pursue my consuming interest in wildlife. My school had an excellent biology department directed by a brilliant and eccentric master, the blood-red Socialist son of a baronet and one of those rare individuals who makes learning a breathtaking excitement. Under him we collected rare leeches that had attached themselves to the bodies of dead dogs floating in the city's derelict canals, cooked (and had to eat) the prime cuts of white mice, and dissected not just rabbits and guinea pigs but also octopuses and giant African snails.

The moors around my home teemed with lizards, hedgehogs, hares, and toads. There were bats in the barns of the old stone Pennine farmhouses and foxes and badgers in the quarries which had supplied the stone that built the farmhouses. It was not merely an interest in biology that motivated me. Beyond the ordered mysteries of the living organism, the deeper fascination for me has always been the capricious, subversive processes of disease and illness.

I spent much of my time out of doors, and I made a point of looking for sick and injured creatures. Armed only with my first book on animal medicine, a small volume intended for pharmacists giving over-the-counter first-aid advice, I scoured the countryside for likely patients. There were plenty of ailing hedgehogs which I would bring in for hospitalization in the garden shed. My simple methods of nursing and giving vitamins and invalid food through eye droppers met with a singular and enduring lack of success but landed me with regular invasions of fleas. On the moors I would frequently find single sheep lying alone, incapable of rising to their feet, and would try to get them going again, but without any understanding of the mechanisms of disease—the underlying calcium deficiency, the septic womb, or the fluke-infested liver—that was at the root of the creature's problems. With my tonics, my vitamins, the small quantities of alcohol that I had removed from my father's liquor cabinet, I would struggle for hours in the rain to achieve my first cure. It was very depressing; an animal never seemed to rally for long as a result of my medical care and I would trudge home rather down at the mouth. But in the morning my enthusiasm would be as unfailing as ever and I would return to the fields with renewed optimism.

With injured birds, the sparrows and starlings that comprised the bulk of my "surgical" practice, I had relatively more success. Tiny limbs with shattered bones could sometimes be restored by devising splints and casts from matchsticks, paper clips, and Scotch tape.

I still count as one of my most satisfying operations

the occasion on which I found a badly injured barn owl and hurried it in for emergency kitchen-table orthopaedics. As usual on such occasions my nurse, anaesthetist (all we had was a freezing spray aerosol), and porter was my grandmother, who would clear the cooking and the pots and pans from the operation table without complaint. The owl had flown into a telegraph wire and had sustained an ugly compound fracture of the major wing bone. It seemed beyond the scope of my matchsticks and tape. At the time I was an avid reader of medical autobiographies, and I was particularly impressed by George Sava's *The Way of a Surgeon*. For the first time I'd read about the mending of human fractures by inserting steel pins inside the marrow cavity. I'd never seen it done or even seen pictures of the technique, but something clicked in my mind. I decided to try to re-join the two pieces of wing bone by slipping something of the right diameter inside the hollow shafts.

The only steel knitting needles in the house were too heavy or too narrow; bits of them wouldn't be any use. Then I had an idea. While grandmother kept a firm grip on the owl and occasionally rechilled the operation site with the aerosol, I went through my collection of birds' feathers. I soon found what I wanted, a stout but light quill from some bird of prey. I cut the quill and sharpened both ends with a knife. After boiling the quill briefly in a pan of water I set to work. The quill fitted perfectly into the exposed marrow cavities, and it didn't take long to fix the fractured segments firmly together. I stitched up the skin wound with needle and cotton and then tested the wing to see how it felt. It seemed solidly intact.

The owl recuperated in the garden shed, and I was kept busy finding field mice and voles for its meals. The wound healed cleanly, and the underlying bone apparently took kindly to the quill pin so fortuitously donated by a fellow hawk or falcon.

At the end of three weeks the owl was able to flap the injured wing very strongly, and I decided to test it out. One evening I took the bird out into the fields and released it. To my great delight it soared off into the twilight sky. That night I lay in bed and grinned happily in the darkness as I heard it hooting away in the woods.

The Scots have a fine reputation in the field of veterinary medicine, and I had always hoped to study for my degree in a Scottish university. When the time came I was enrolled by Glasgow University, where I was graduated after five years. The first thing I did was to marry Shelagh, a girl from my home town whom I had been courting since my first year in veterinary school. She was a radiographer working on the therapy of malignancies by X-ray and radioactive isotopes. There were some advantageous spin-offs for my work when I met Shelagh, a principal one being the way in which she would cooperate in smuggling suitably doped dogs and cats with inoperable cancers into her hospital department during lunch hours so that I could try out some clandestine irradiation of the malignancies.

After qualifying in 1956, I decided to stay on in Glasgow for a course in comparative pathology. It was a far-sighted move which still benefits me today, for much of the investigation of disease in exotic animals depends on the proper handling, examination, and interpretation of specimens of diseased tissue, on microscopic work, and on the bacteriological testing of samples of blood, pus, and other liquids.

After one year of this I went back to my home town of Rochdale to join a general practice dealing with a wide range of large and small animals. It was the firm with which I had been associated during vacations as a student, and which had as a client the large Belle Vue Zoo in Manchester, twelve miles away. I would be able to work with exotic animals as well as receiving a sound grounding in all aspects of general veterinary work.

There could not have been a better place for a young vet to practice. Stitching and cutting, injecting and lancing, struggling to replace the prolapsed womb of a cow on a Pennine farm at three o'clock on a blizzard-swept February morning, digging up rotten carcasses of pigs to obtain pancreas glands for hog cholera tests, pinning stray tomcats' fractured limbs just after closing time on Saturday nights, delicately removing fatty tumours as big as plums from parrots with beaks that could slice steel—it was the finest training.

That, too, is something I'm grateful for today, for the art of surgery is the same whether it is performed on a pig or a panda, a lamb or a llama. Everything I learned on domestic animals about handling animal tissues, opening and closing limbs and organs, using drugs, and handling violent, awkward, and terrified creatures could be applied to wild animals. Surgery is, after all, just needlework; the more you learn to cut and stitch confidently and neatly, the better you become. Likewise, it is by his work on the obstetric problems of cows, dogs, and horses that a vet must acquire his skill in correcting a baby's position manually within the womb and in performing Caesarean operations. There are just not enough cases of complicated births occurring in giraffes or polar bears for him to refine his techniques by working on those species alone.

I had been in general practice for almost nine years when one day Ray Legge, the director of the Belle Vue Zoo, said something about it being "understandably the usual practice" for zoos to call in doctors of human medicine when their great apes were ill. The statement struck a nerve in me. Of course it was understandable in some ways: great apes—gorillas, orang-utans, and chimpanzees—do resemble man in many respects and have similar disease problems. However, these doctors never seemed to treat cases of disease in the great apes quite seriously enough. We had had lots of co-operation from medical workers at places such as Manchester University, but when it came down to it they were interested mainly in their own speciality—the ophthalmologists were keen to get specimens for their collections of retinas or lenses, the anaesthetists were happy to try out new hypnotics, the virologists wanted blood serum and more blood serum for their comparative studies. All well and good, but none of them was interested or cared deeply enough for the animals themselves, as individual patients with problems to be cured.

I decided that it was time for someone in the veterinary profession to show that the medicine of great apes was a serious veterinary field. To that end I decided to study for the Fellowship of the Royal College of Veterinary Surgeons in Diseases of Zoo Primates.

It wasn't easy. Working in the practice with visits during the morning, operations in the afternoon, and consulting hours at night, I found it difficult to make time for study. I bombarded myself with facts and figures during my waking hours by covering the walls of the bathroom, kitchen, dining room, and lounge in my house with big pieces of paper on which were boldly printed lists of things that I must learn. Every recorded parasite of each species of monkey or ape, together with its life cycle, symptoms and treatment, minute details of the various types of brain disease that can affect these creatures, and a thousand and one other items were emblazoned in prominent positions

above the television set, over the fireplace, and directly opposite the toilet seat. The classification and characteristics
of the various monkey malaria microbes were crayoned
around the faces of the clocks and in the center of the telephone dials. The house was awash with paper. It was impossible to get away from facts. Learn them I had to and
learn them I did. Even Shelagh and my two daughters
were subliminally indoctrinated by the welter of paper
information; to this day both Stephanie and Lindsey can
recite a complete list of tapeworms to be found in the
lower bowel of rhesus monkeys.

On my half-days off I worked at the great ape house
in Belle Vue or pored over books in the Medical Library at
the University. On weekends I travelled round the British
zoos such as Twycross and Regent's Park, which have extensive primate collections. I made the most of every
photographer's monkey or circus chimp that came my
way during surgery hours. Eventually, after a long written
examination in Glasgow and a practical and oral examination at the Edinburgh Zoo, I obtained my FRCVS. To
celebrate, Shelagh and I bought a Japanese bronze of a
mother tortoise and her brood, and I went off to my first
big international symposium on zoo animal diseases in
Austria.

I also made up my mind to leave general practice and
see if I could earn a living purely from exotic animals.
Would I be able to build up the contacts and experience so
far achieved into a full independent livelihood?

If I was going to do it I must do it properly. No more
dogs or cats or pigs or cattle. I would set up an office at my
home just outside Rochdale and accept nothing but calls
concerning exotic animal cases. It was a gamble. Like all
vets I am bound by rules of professional conduct, so it was
not possible to advertise my presence, and snakes and mon-

keys and parrots are much, much thinner on the ground in Lancashire than are dogs and ponies. Nor is there much in the way of fees when treating sore eyes in a child's three-inch terrapin or replacing the prolapsed anus of a six-inch grass snake.

Those first few weeks after I severed my ties with my old general practice were not particularly cheerful. On the one hand, I was constantly on the telephone turning down clients with domestic or farm animals who could not understand that I would not in future be dealing with their sort of animal. On the other, the hoped-for influx of parrot and lizard and monkey owners did not materialize. I circularized all the veterinary practices in the area, informing them that I was no longer working with domestic animals and stating that I was prepared to see any exotic cases which they might care to send my way; all that resulted was a stream of telephone calls from veterinarians asking for advice about the small reptiles or unusual species of birds in their surgeries whose owners were unwilling to travel fifty or perhaps a hundred miles to Rochdale for specialist attention. I was going to be hard put to make a living. The plain fact was that exotic pets in general have a low cash value. It is cheaper to replace them than to cart them about the country just to see some vet who is interested in their particular complaint.

All was not gloom, however. From time to time a lion cub or a chimpanzee would appear at the back door. An old lady with a dearly loved red patas monkey would cram it into a plastic box and push it on a trolley for three or four miles up the lane to see me. Every six weeks or so a jolly gentleman in a Rolls-Royce would pull up, and I would go out to examine the sick and ill-tempered puma that was irritably chewing up the fine leather of the back seat. When that was over I would examine the hawk which

perched hooded and immobile on the automatic gearshift.
The jolly gentleman would finally open the trunk of the car
and unwind fifteen feet of python for my inspection.

Most important, I had kept Belle Vue Zoo as a client,
and my duties there were satisfyingly diversified and sometimes even tinged with drama. A few episodes from that
time still stand out in my mind.

For example, there was the time a new hippopotamus,
Hercules, arrived at Belle Vue from Whipsnade Zoo. He
had been shipped in a massive crate made out of thick
wooden beams reinforced with steel bands, for the hippo
is not a creature to be trifled with. It can hurl itself forward or spin round on its hind feet with remarkable agility,
it is as unstoppable as a tank, and it delivers a fearsome
chomping, crushing bite. To be on the safe side, Whipsnade
had given Hercules a dose of phencyclidine before sending him off and had strongly recommended that he should
receive a further shot just before he was uncrated in Manchester. They feared that otherwise an irascible hippo
might emerge and make his way like an express train, walls
and so on notwithstanding, towards the city centre.

Hercules' crate was open-topped, and by climbing up
the side I could look down on his steaming armour-plating.
He was standing calmly enough and showed little sign of
the effects of the sedative. I had not unloaded a hippo before. My inclination would have been to forgo the second
phencyclidine injection, but Whipsnade, with much more
experience of these matters at the time, had made the point
strongly. They had even sent a measured dose of the drug.

I filled a syringe, bent down over the side of the crate,
and slapped my stoutest needle through the hippo's rump.
Hercules reacted by slamming my wrist hard against the
wooden side of the crate. I was trapped securely. Hercules
maintained the pressure against my wrist with all his might.

He wiggled his hips a bit and ground my hand excruciatingly into the wood. Biting my tongue, I slapped vainly at the hippo's bottom with my other hand. It was some minutes before he pulled away and I was allowed to retrieve my extremity, now numb, black, and horribly scuffed. I still have no feeling in that part of my wrist.

After a quarter of an hour Hercules was still standing, but his ears were drooping slightly and there was a string of saliva hanging from his jaw. I decided to let him out. The bolts were removed from the reinforced rear door and the door itself was opened wide. We wanted to make him back out so that he would be less likely to charge. Hercules did not budge. No matter what we did, tapping his nose with a stick, tempting him with food, or slapping his back, he would not go into reverse gear. So we cautiously opened the front door and gazed on his bucolic features for the first time.

Hercules stared blandly at the inside of the tropical river house where he was now to live, sniffed disdainfully, and blinked his drowsy eyelids. Then he saw the shining pool of warm water before him, its surface wreathed in misty vapour. Very sedately he began to move forward. He emerged from the crate, paused briefly, then walked slowly towards the pool. He went down the ramp at the side of the pool as if on tiptoe, sniffed at the water, found it to his liking, and gracefully slipped in. Through the clear water we could see him settle peacefully on the bottom of the pool.

A cluster of icicles formed in the pit of my stomach. "It looks as if he's going to sleep," I told the keepers around me. "Get some ropes, fast. We could be in big trouble!"

The second dose of phencyclidine, together with the soothing warm bath, was having a potentially lethal effect. A conscious hippo can hold its breath underwater for many minutes but will eventually come to the surface to take in a fresh gulp of air. A doped hippo might very well be a different matter. Suppose Hercules inhaled blissfully while dreaming on the bottom of his pool?

Some of the men dashed off. The zoo director and I stood at the water's edge looking anxiously down at the recumbent form of the hippo, his head three feet below the surface. When the ropes arrived there was only one thing for it. Stripping to our underpants, the head keeper, Matt Kelly, and I jumped into the water and dived for the submerged hulk. It is no easy task to feel one's way over a hippo's anatomy without the benefit of a pair of goggles while towing a length of thick rope. Spluttering, we both surfaced for a quick discussion on a plan of action.

"You try to get a rope on the back legs, Matt," I said. "I'll see if I can get one round the neck."

Matt dived again and I followed. Hercules slumbered on, unaware of the visitors struggling clumsily about his submarine bedroom. I would not have dared to take such liberties with a hippo in full possession of its senses.

After much effort and repeated returns to the surface with bursting lungs, we managed to place the ropes more or less as we wanted them. The keepers hauled mightily and to my relief Hercules, most un-Venus-like, rose to the surface. The great nostrils opened as his head cleared the water, and he exhaled gently. His eyes were half closed and there was a pleasant softening of the hippo's usual grim smile.

It was impossible to drag the heavy creature onto land. There were not enough of us, hippos have no convenient handles, and I was afraid that excessive use of ropes on Hercules' limbs and neck might injure him. In water he weighed much less. We would have to support him in the pool by passing ropes under his belly until he was no longer under the influence. We kept his head up by wrapping towels round it and slinging it to a beam. Hercules looked for all the world as if he was suffering an attack of toothache and had taken to the whisky bottle to alleviate the pain.

After some hours Hercules began to wriggle on the supporting ropes. His eyes opened fully and he surveyed the strange scene sombrely. When he realized that his towel bandage inhibited chomping, he became restless and we decided that he had come round enough to look after himself. After being untangled he retired to the bottom of the pool, from which secure position he looked up at us lugubriously. Several minutes later I watched him come to the surface to breathe deeply. Hercules was going to be all right.

Hercules was indeed all right. He immediately fell in love with his pool, which was set in an imitation tropical jungle with waterfalls, islands, and luscious vegetation. His arrival, however, spelt disaster for some other denizens of the Manchester jungle. Sharing his habitat were tapirs, capybaras, and an assortment of exotic birds. These Hercules proceeded to stalk and, if possible, eat. He would play the crocodile, lurking beneath the surface of the water, now dark with his droppings, and using his protuberant eyes as mini-periscopes. When a tapir came down to drink or a bird perched on a rock at the water's edge, Hercules would glide stealthily in like a killer submarine. With a sudden charge when he was within inches of his prey, he would seize it in his jaws, kill it instantly with one powerful crunch, and feast until not a scrap remained. So much for vegetarianism: Hercules fancied meat. He still does. Sometimes when he is off-colour I stand on the rocks by his pool and toss him loaves packed with pick-me-ups or stimulants. I have to watch carefully for a pair of gleaming eyes that just about break the water surface and come slowly but steadily towards my feet. At such moments I skip smartly backwards.

Another incident I remember, not so much for what did happen as for what could have happened, is the morning Adam, the male orang-utan, escaped from the great ape house. It was the height of summer and Adam had gone to visit Miniland, an exhibition of miniature fairy-tale villages and model tableaux from children's stories. When I arrived, he was sitting on the partly demolished cathedral of Notre Dame chewing the leg off the hunchback. He gazed at us blandly as he chewed. I approached him slowly, accompanied by Len, his keeper. Len talked soothingly to him; he had looked after the orang since it was the size of a cat. How were we to get Adam back into his quarters? This was before the first dart-guns became available in Britain. I had phencyclidine in my bag but how was I going to administer it?

Adam threw the mutilated torso of the hunchback at us and grimaced threateningly. He shuffled truculently off, pausing only to pick up one of the Three Bears and knock down Don Quixote's windmill with it. Then he made for the open spaces of the zoo gardens; he did not even glance back at us as he lolloped smoothly over the ground. Len, head keeper Matt Kelly, the zoo director, and I followed anxiously. A mature orang-utan is immensely powerful, as Len had reason to know; an orang had recently sunk its teeth through his shoe and bitten off one of his toes. Adam might cause panic among the visitors. He had the muscular power of three full-grown men. What if he grabbed hold of a child?

Fortunately Adam, like most orang-utans, was a shy and undemonstrative creature, without the brash exhibitionism of the chimpanzee or the mercurial changes in mood of the gorilla. As he wandered across the flower beds, now trailing an umbrella borrowed firmly but without physical violence from an astounded passerby, he spied a small wooden hut used by the gardeners and went in and started to vandalize the interior.

At least he was confined. We crept up to the door and bolted it. Adam was too busy smashing plant pots to notice us.

What now? We sat outside and waited and discussed the matter. Len looked at his watch. "It's almost eleven o'clock," he said. "It's his soup time."

When I had taken over the care of the animals at Belle Vue Zoo I had introduced the feeding of plenty of meat to the great apes. Best pig's liver, chicken, and mincemeat were given daily. Animal protein of this kind is essential for the apes' complete health, and indeed it has produced a remarkable increase in the length and glossiness of their coats. All the meat is cooked to avoid risk of infection, and the left-over gravy, with added vegetables, herbs, and cereals, is made into a soup which is given to the animals at eleven o'clock as a mid-morning pick-me-up. The apes seem to appreciate it greatly.

"Can you put some dope in the soup?" Len went on. "He'll probably take it."

It was a good idea. Len went off to fetch the warm broth while I measured out a dose of phencyclidine with a syringe. Adam's bright orange eyes watched us through the hut's small window. When Len returned I took the mug of soup and went round to the windowless rear of the hut, away from those orange eyes, and mixed in the sedative. I went back and gave the mug to Len.

Adam was now sitting on a pile of shattered plant pots by the window. His stomach told him it was time for elevenses. Len pushed the window open and passed the mug through. Most politely Adam took his soup and drank it, smacking his lips and licking the mug dry as far as his tongue could reach. We watched and waited. Slowly but surely the great ape's upper eyelids became heavy. He began to drool a thin thread of saliva and his lower lip sagged. In ten minutes he was asleep and then we carried him, like some pot-bellied and surfeited potentate, back to his house.

Len played a part in yet another episode that remains vividly in my memory. This time it involved Jo-Jo, the gorilla. I had tended Jo-Jo and Suzy, who was to become his mate, from the time they first arrived in Manchester as young babies. Gorilla infants are notoriously delicate and easily succumb to human germs. We took every precaution to give them a strong and healthy start, including putting a ban on taking any of the great apes out of the zoo to children's parties, fêtes, and the like. That cut out the major source of flu, colds, and infantile ailments. Using glass walls instead of bars for the heated indoor compartments in the ape house also played a significant part in preventing the spread of bacteria and viruses from the public to the animals. All the keeping staff were regularly vaccinated against influenza and screened for tuberculosis. Special measures were taken against cockroaches, a frequent visitor to animal houses, which can carry poliomyelitis. Like children, Jo-Jo and Suzy also had polio vaccine on lumps of sugar. The air in their sleeping quarters was filtered and treated with anti-fungal chemicals, and their fruit and vegetables were washed to remove traces of any pesticide or other substance sprayed on by the grower.

As their keeper, Len virtually lived with Jo-Jo and

Suzy in a small room nearby in the ape house. There he would prepare their special diet, measure out their vitamin drops, boil their milk and slip in a nourishing egg, whip up their Ovaltine nightcap, and select the ingredients for their broth from a larder plentifully stocked with vegetables of all kinds from asparagus and leeks to string beans and black-eyed peas. Len also spent long periods playing with and nursing the little creatures, a very important part of his job. Their games were simple and boisterous: playing tag, wrestling, somersaulting. The animals thrived and grew rapidly and our precautions seemed to work well.

Jo-Jo soon grew into a powerful young juvenile who packed quite a punch when playing with humans. Suzy was gentler and more reticent, but Jo-Jo liked nothing better than his daily roustabouts with Len, Matt Kelly, or the zoo director, Ray Legge. His favourite wheeze was to saunter past one's legs, apparently intent on other business and ignoring one's presence. But as he drew level he would deliver a beefy clout to the kneecap with a flick of his hand and scurry off gleefully, looking back over his shoulder for the expected pursuit. The bigger he got the more the kneecaps, mine included, began to complain.

The gorillas loved being picked up and cuddled. This was easy when they weighed ten or twenty pounds, but muscular seventy-pound youngsters who insisted on being rocked in one's arms were more of a problem. The trouble was not the ache in the arms as the ape lay dozing cheek to cheek but the crucial point when the nursing and playing had to stop until the next day. Like spoilt children Jo-Jo and Suzy objected petulantly to being left to their own devices and would nip firmly at bits of human anatomy or seize hold of clothing with a vise-like grip. At first they were not big enough to enforce their point of view too vigorously, but as time went on this behaviour made inspections increasingly more tricky. I would go into their indoor quarters with Ray Legge and Len. To have a good look at Jo-Jo's gums, to see whether his colour was satisfactory, to peer with an ophthalmoscope into his dark and sparkling eyes, or to listen to his chest with a stethoscope meant first playing the kneecap-knocking game and then, when I could stand no more, letting my playmate drape himself around me for a cuddle. When he was satisfactorily positioned in my arms with bits of him looped round my neck, poked into my ear, or lovingly entangled with my hair, I would use a free arm if I had one, or someone else's if not, to remove the necessary instrument from my pocket and place it surreptitiously on the appropriate spot. The examination over, I then had to rid myself of the gorilla, which meant passing him to somebody else, usually Len. Neither gorilla minded being swapped in this way, seeming to think one cuddler as good as another. Len would then be the last to leave the quarters. After Ray Legge and I had gone, Len would detach the gorilla from his person and put him on the floor. As the animal began to protest and grab for him again, Len would slip quickly out through the door.

That was how it was at first, but as time went on Len did not always make it. He would find himself squeezing dexterously through the door into the passage with two, three, or four shiny black arms reattaching themselves to his clothing, limbs, or hair. Increasingly he left bits behind, and the rigmarole of breaking off the day's fun became longer and more complex.

Came the day when the three of us were in the gorilla quarters for my routine medical inspection, and Jo-Jo, now developing the auburn shock of hair on his forehead characteristic of a mature male and rippling his biceps like Mr. Universe, decided on a showdown.

Jo-Jo's examination went without any trouble. He clung to me with an innocent expression on his face and snuffled at my ear. Then it was time to leave him. As soon as I nonchalantly tried to set him down I felt his muscles tighten. He bared his teeth and lost his innocent look.

"You'd better have him as usual," I told Len.

Len came alongside and Jo-Jo thought about it. OK, he was prepared to move across. Seventy pounds of warm and hairy gorilla slipped from my arms with movements like mercury and made itself comfortable round Len's upper half. As usual, Ray Legge and I left the room and Len backed off towards the door. Once there he tried to unpick the ape, but either Jo-Jo's grip got tighter or the hold was simply transferred to another part of Len's anatomy. As soon as Len managed to free one hand from his shoulder, its place would be taken by a foot or, more menacingly, by a strong pair of jaws digging in not quite hard enough to break the skin but with a mouthful of flesh securely imprisoned. Len struggled and cajoled. Titbits of grapes and bananas and apricots were brought. Jo-Jo was not to be bought off. If Len was leaving the room, so was Jo-Jo; the gorilla seemed determined to maintain the Siamese-twin relationship forever.

"Let me have a go with him," said Ray Legge. "Perhaps he'll let me put him down. Anyway, I'm perhaps a bit more nimble than you, Len."

He went back in. Yes, Jo-Jo was quite happy about another change. The look of innocence returned to his face as he transferred his affections to the zoo director. Now it was Ray Legge's turn to move with his burden until he was just inside the door and then, cooing soothingly and stroking Jo-Jo's head with one hand, try to loosen the ape's hold with his other hand. Nothing doing. Jo-Jo stuck like a malevolent limpet. He pretended to be snoozing peacefully but his iron-hard black nails dug into the zoo director's clothing with a sudden sharp movement. I swear he was peeping out between closed eyelids.

Half an hour went by and it was time to try another change. Matt Kelly was called in. Jo-Jo went to him like a lamb, but when Matt tried to divest himself of the animal he lost some hair, a pocket, and all the buttons from his shirt front, but he did not lose the gorilla.

I was in a quandary. Transferring the gorilla was easy, but at this rate we would soon run out of gorilla holders. Dope seemed to be the answer, but the prick of a tranquillizing injection might stimulate Jo-Jo to take it out on the current holder before dropping off to sleep, and gorillas can bite hard and rip viciously with their fingers. We would have to do it without inflicting even a minute amount of pain, which meant that the only way to administer the drug was by mouth. In the food store I injected a knock-out dose of phencyclidine into the pulp of a banana without actually peeling the fruit. Jo-Jo likes to peel his own.

Back in the ape house Matt was sitting glumly on the floor, almost totally submerged by the loving heap of gorilla that clasped him. There is a rule about giving doped bananas to apes or doctored sausages to wolves or hollowed-out loaves of bread containing medicine to suspicious hippopotamuses: Always proffer first a sterling, pristine, untampered-with, impeccable article of the same kind. Having established your credentials with number one, you then emerge in your true colours by doing the dirty on number two.

With this in mind I offered a normal banana to Jo-Jo. He took it, peeled it with one hand and his teeth (the other hand was maintaining its hold on Matt's right ear), ate the pulp with relish, licked the skin, and threw it down.

Now I produced the Trojan horse, or rather the Trojan banana. Again Jo-Jo took it, peeled it, and prepared to thrust it into his mouth. Then out of the recesses of his mind came either a generous thought or, more likely I suspect, an inkling, just an embryonic inkling, that malpractice was afoot. With a gentle pouting of his lips and a soothing cooing sound, Jo-Jo rammed the fruit of the banana firmly between Matt's lips. The head keeper spluttered and gulped, but Jo-Jo was insistent that Matt was going to have his banana. I was horrified. If Matt swallowed the doctored banana pulp he would be unconscious within ten minutes and, worse, might suffer for days afterwards from the side effects reported in humans of erotic fantasies and burning sensations in the extremities.

"Spit it out, for God's sake!" I howled. "Don't swallow any banana, Matt!"

Matt spat for dear life. Jo-Jo seemed distinctly surprised at his ingratitude and tried to poke bits of the mushed pulp back between Matt's teeth. Matt continued to puff out furiously, rolling his eyes at us as we stood watching helplessly. Suzy came over and helped clean up the mess. She picked the spat-out bits off Jo-Jo's hairy chest like a wife carefully sponging soup stains off her husband's dinner jacket. Not a bit of the banana did Jo-Jo eat, nor would he accept any further pieces of food.

Eventually, for it was by now well on into the evening, we tried to relieve poor Matt by doing yet another change, this time back to Len again. The transfer went smoothly, but still Len could not get out of the room without his ape.

At last it was decided to leave Len in the gorilla quarters. A comfortable chair was brought in and a transistor radio was left playing outside the door. When Ray Legge went back at midnight Jo-Jo was still comfortably, immovably, *in situ*. Len was trying to doze. It was seven o'clock the following morning before Jo-Jo finally fell into a deep, forgetful slumber and Len was able to lower him gently to the floor, steal out of the room, and lock up.

Never again have we gone in with the two gorillas. They are now adult, and when I need to examine them I use the dart-gun and a tranquillizer. But we all remember affectionately the happy times we had playing tag when they were babies. Like children, it's a pity they have to grow up.

3 The Whistling Pumas

During the uncertain days following my decision to limit my practice to the treatment of exotic animals, Shelagh's buoyancy and optimism kept my own spirits up and reinforced my belief that I had made the right decision. She cleaned out and wallpapered the small dairy attached to the stone Jacobean farmhouse which is our home, covered the floor with rubberized tiles, ran up some colourful curtains on her sewing machine, and turned a set of elegant curtain rails and brackets on the lathe at the Wednesday evening woodwork classes. The end-product was a comfortable office-*cum*-examination room for me.

Shelagh was also indispensable to the practice itself. We had a wooden hut built in the market garden to house sick and injured big cats, which Shelagh nursed after treatment until they were fully recovered. Quite a string of animals came through our house for this sort of special attention. The first occupant for the wooden hut was a paralysed male lion cub that had been bitten by his father. One of the lion's teeth had penetrated to the cub's spinal cord, setting up an abscess, and the cub was unable to control the functions of his rear end. I operated on him on the kitchen table, cutting down to the infected area of bone, draining it, and releasing pressure on the big nerve.

Then Shelagh took over, cleaning him up several times a day and protecting his bottom from painful "scalding" by meticulous washing and the application of baby oil. Eventually the cub regained the use of his legs and developed into a strong and normal animal.

An orphan wallaby came to us that was only three inches long. Shelagh reared it, setting the alarm clock for hourly feeds with an eye dropper throughout the day and night. In the daytime, by carrying the pink, hairless creature in a home-made flannel pouch slung round her waist beneath her clothing against the comforting warmth of her stomach, she was able to do her housework in a fashion. At night, in the sixty-minute periods between each feed, she would try to catch forty winks by sleeping upright in a chair with a pouch still in its usual position.

One evening we went out to dinner at a nearby restaurant. As the soup was being ladled out, Shelagh felt the baby wallaby awaken and start to wriggle. She thrust her hand down her waistband and pulled out the struggling little marsupial, all bright eyes and flailing limbs, under the astounded gaze of the head waiter. "Ah—are you all right, madam?" he spluttered, pouring a portion of minestrone onto the tablecloth. I'm sure he believed he was witnessing a remarkably unexpected miscarriage being undergone by a most nonchalant mother-to-be. I reassured the poor fellow, and after pointing out that the "no dogs allowed" rule of the dining room made no mention of wallabies, we got on with the business of eye-dropping warm milk into the baby from the small Thermos flask Shelagh carried in her bag. Then, having repacked the now-contented infant back under her skirt, we continued with our own repast.

After the wallaby rearing came two more orphans, a pair of puma twins. We did not know it at the time, but their advent was to trigger a crucial watershed in my career.

One of the perennial problems of all zoos and safari parks, particularly the urban ones, is the unwelcome arrival of domestic cats, which prowl around the grounds looking for scraps of food. These scavengers transmit potentially lethal diseases to the exotic animals. Cat influenza and a serious liver disease, panleucopenia, originate from their nocturnal visits and from their habit of leaving excrement and marking their territories in urine in places where the zoo animals will go during the daytime. In the morning when the big cats are released from their night houses, they sniff at their visitors' souvenirs, inhaling active virus particles of diseases that are the greatest menaces to captive cats.

Something like this happened to one female puma (known as a cougar or a mountain lion in the United States) who was heavily pregnant and expected to deliver her cubs within a few days' time. Like the other cats in the zoo she had been vaccinated and regularly boosted against panleucopenia infection, but as sometimes happens in pregnant animals the period of gestation had been accompanied by a fall in resistance to certain infections, and one night, when the big cats were all in their sleeping quarters and the keepers had gone home, the expectant mother became suddenly very ill. No one was around to observe the first signs of trouble or note that the animal's soaring rise in temperature had begun to induce labour. With her circulation faltering and the heart's pumping action becoming alarmingly irregular under the onslaught of the virus, two little spotted, coffee-coloured cubs were born. Eyes closed, protesting with puny squeaks, and scrabbling instinctively with soggy boneless feet at the placental membranes surrounding them, they managed to free themselves partially and draw in fitfully the first air of their lives. There was no one to help them, no abrasive tongue to clean the mucus off their coats and get them stirring, no one to cut the few inches of umbilical cord that linked them firmly to the placenta still retained in the mother's birth canal. The acute virus attack and the stress of giving birth was too much for the female puma. Before the two cubs could be completely freed and the act of birth properly terminated, the puma became unconscious, stopped breathing, and died.

When the keeper went into the big cat house the following morning he found the two cubs, weak and chilled, still attached to the tissue within their lifeless mother. Cutting the cords with his penknife, the keeper rubbed the little creatures briskly between his hands, stuffed them under his pullover, and ran for the phone, hoping that the shaking up and the warmth of his body would begin to revive them while he summoned help.

Half an hour later I arrived at the zoo and for the first time set eyes on the two scraps of fur that we were later to call Morecambe and Wise, after two celebrated English comedy stars. Their temperature was still subnormal after the night's contact with a cold concrete floor. Their movements were lethargic. They were voiceless, opening their mouths to protest as I examined them but too weak to produce any noise. I used my preferred method of revival, which has produced the most success for me with a succession of cubs from polar bears and wolves to cheetahs, leopards, and tigers. Gripping their tiny hind legs firmly, I whirled them around my head, using centrifugal force to drain the sticky mucus from their minute windpipes and bronchi. Then I dunked them in a bowl of water, heated to just higher than body temperature, and alternated the dunkings with brisk rubbings with a coarse dry towel. I dropped concentrated sugar solution into their mouths and injected them with stimulants for the breathing and circulation systems. Gradually the lilac colour of their tongues and the roofs of their mouths changed to a healthier pink, and instead of lying in my hands like flaccid lumps of putty, a more spring-like tension returned to their muscles and they began to right themselves more vigorously when held upside down. At last they produced audible squeaks.

I asked the zoo director what he intended to do with them, for I knew pumas are not especially prized as zoo animals—they breed rather easily and hence their value is low.

"Well," he said, "I'm afraid they wouldn't be worth the trouble and expense of bringing up. We wouldn't get as much for them as they will cost in milk alone. And we've enough full-grown and immature pumas on the place as it is. I'm afraid that it might be best for you to put them down."

I looked at the scraps of scrabbling fur lying in the palms of my hands. I have always been more of a cat than a dog man. The aesthetics, the life-style, the elegance, the poise, the independence, and the lack of servility of all species of the cat family strongly appeal to me. Cats are good to feel, great to watch, funny or fearsome, and always decorative. Shelagh is even more of a cat fanatic than I. I couldn't destroy these two little beginners, nor could I go home and tell my wife that I had done so. I decided to rear the cubs myself—or, rather, I decided to ask Shelagh to take on the task.

I put the two cubs in a cardboard box with a hot water bottle and then rang home. "Can't talk long, I've got to get home as soon as I can," I said. "I've got two little orphans for you to raise. Clear out the little library under the stairs, we're going to have pumas!" Quite used to terse messages of this kind at all hours of the day and night, Shelagh, I knew, would be ready with all the necessary gear by the time I got home.

So it began. The cubs were installed in the warm

library and cosseted in every possible way. To begin with, they were kept in a cardboard box lined with a blanket and were fed twice hourly on Carnation milk. After each feed we rubbed them briskly with a bit of dry towel, trying to imitate the rough licking of a mother puma's tongue, in the hope that this would produce by reflex action a satisfying emptying of the minute bowels and bladders.

The cubs thrived. It was amazing how quickly they grew. After a couple of weeks they were able to climb out of the cardboard box and then, neither of them obviously being of a literary bent, they adamantly persisted in trudging out of the book room and seeking refuge behind the high iron grate inside the living room fireplace. They gradually learned to lap their food, which we slowly and progressively thickened, first with beaten egg and later with pureed raw steak. They were immaculately clean. From the very beginning they caught on to the purpose of a piece of newspaper set down in a particular place in the living room. There they would crouch, rigid as statues, to answer the call of nature, their eyes watering with concentration. When sometimes, particularly as they grew older, the volume of waste threatened to spill over on to the carpet, Shelagh would change the newspaper while the puma was still in mid-operation. With one hand she would lift up the crouching cat, which would remain in a frozen sphinx-like posture within her grasp and continue to stare fixedly into the distance. With the other hand she deftly exchanged the soiled sheet for a clean one. During such transfer operations the outflow of waste from the appropriate exits was always obligingly suspended, to be resumed only when the seemingly cataleptic cub was safely plonked onto the clean paper.

Morecambe and Wise were wonderfully attractive.

Like all young pumas they were spotted, with outsize ears and paws a few sizes too big for them. When alarmed they hissed and spat, but when they were in a friendly mood, or calling either to one another or to us, they emitted charming birdlike whistles. In fact, the cubs showed some ability to charm birds with their music. They would sit gazing out of the window that overlooks our front garden and trill away merrily at the birds that hopped out on the lawn or fished for snails in the little pond. Sure enough, after the two cubs had been serenading for a few minutes, a blackbird or a thrush would fly up onto the window ledge outside. As the bird turned its head quizzically to the pane of glass, the young pumas would flatten their damp noses hard against the glass and sing joyously on.

But the animals grew apace, and gradually the house began to show the effects. Their favourite hidey-hole inside the fireplace was becoming too small for them, and their efforts to pack in their plump and muscular bodies were beginning to dislodge the iron grate and the copper hood suspended above it. All slippers belonging to members of the family had been eaten, Shelagh's nylons enjoyed a life expectancy of approximately fifteen minutes, and Morecambe had learned how to open the refrigerator door. We noticed that friends didn't call as often, and they certainly never brought their pet dogs with them any more. A visiting poodle or fox terrier just couldn't take the nerve-shattering experience of ambling into an apparently empty room with its owner, to find itself suddenly under gleeful attack by two whooping, whistling, spotted creatures springing from the darkness beyond the hearth. The Electricity Board meter men took to sending estimated accounts, and representatives of drug firms seemed increasingly to opt for pushing their promotional literature into the mail box instead of coming in to discuss new

products. Sadly, Shelagh and I realized that the time had
come for Morecambe and Wise to go to somewhere more
suitable for their upbringing.

The problem we faced is one which inevitably con-
fronts all owners of exotic pet animals. Things are great
while the chimpanzee or the monkey or the leopard or
the tiger or the bear is young and cuddlesome, but these
creatures grow far faster than human infants and, particularly as they approach sexual maturity, become unpredictable in their behaviour. The muscle power of an adult
monkey, the mature teeth and claws of the big cats, the
need to provide adequate space for exercise, the increasing
requirements in food, and the psychological effects of prolonged contact with humans produce a host of problems.
At this point many owners feel that the day can be saved
by simply going along to the people at the local zoo and
asking them to give a good home to their pet. Sadly, it is
rarely as simple as that.

On the one hand it is hard on the animal, which has
been used to the close confines of the family environment
and has probably never seen another member of its species
since the earliest days of its life. It is completely unpre-
pared psychologically for the zoo or safari park life-style.
What is more, its fellows in the zoo are usually already
organized into social groups which do not readily accept
the odd-ball outsider suddenly thrust upon them. Rarely
can a pet-reared exotic animal be reintroduced happily into
free association with others of its kind. If attempted, it
often ends in the new arrival's being brutally assaulted and
sometimes killed. On other occasions, as with chimps, the
move may appear at first to succeed, but later profound
psychological ill effects will be noticed. Breeding will not
occur because human-fixated, family-reared chimps seem
to lose normal sex drive and either do not mate at all or go

about it in perverted and eventually fruitless ways. Go behind the scenes at many zoos and you will find sad rows of cages, each filled with a single specimen of a particular species, a pet which grew too big for its human owners, which cannot be mixed with zoo stock and which now languishes in sad, solitary confinement, all but forgotten, an indictment of those who first brought it up and then couldn't carry it through.

I was determined that we would return Morecambe and Wise to the zoo before such a stage was reached with them and raised the matter with the director of Belle Vue. Although their monetary value was virtually nil, I asked him to make all efforts to find a home for the two pumas. He promised to do his best, and after a few days he telephoned me to say that he had managed to place them with the Flamingo Park Zoo, in the picturesque vale of Pickering about a hundred miles away. It was a sad day when the Belle Vue van called to take the two cubs over to Yorkshire. Shelagh was near to tears as the vehicle pulled away. Although she couldn't see them, she could hear them whistling apprehensively to her, and she vowed to visit them regularly in their new home to check up on their well being.

A week later we set out to Flamingo Park on our first visit. I had been there only once before. A nilgai antelope had escaped from its sister zoo at Stanley in County Durham, and the director of Flamingo Park, who also controlled Stanley, had asked me to see if I could recapture the animal. The nilgai had been living on the land for about three months, and although numerous reports of its whereabouts had been flowing into Flamingo Park, by the time the keepers arrived on the scene the escapee was always long gone. Eventually it teamed up with a docile herd of

cattle, and although it would not go in for milking with
them at night, it grazed with them during the day.

Approaching a nilgai is an extremely difficult job.
This biggest of all the antelopes has an acute sense of vision
and hearing, and at the slightest hint of anything out of the
ordinary in its surroundings, its powerful muscles can send
it across the countryside, clearing walls and hedges with
ease.

To get to the farm where the nilgai had been reported, I drove for four hours diagonally across north-east
England. I carried with me the only knock-out drug which
I had at that time, phencyclidine, and a dart-gun with a
range of only thirty feet. It was a wet and misty day, and
I remember thinking as I drove through the mining villages of Durham that it would be just my luck for the animal to have moved on once again, and I would miss my
chance of doing my stuff for what might become a new
client.

Once arrived at the scene, I was informed that the
nilgai was still on the premises, grazing somewhere among
the cattle scattered over a pasture that seemed to stretch
on forever, broken here and there by hillocks, hedges,
dense copses, and low-lying boggy areas. The zoo director,
Mr. Bloom, had a plan. A long line of men, keepers from
Flamingo Park and Stanley Zoo, augmented by local farm-
workers and off-duty miners, would walk slowly across
the pasture, hoping to drive the cattle together with the
nilgai in an un-panicked group through a gateway at one
corner. By the gateway was a low stone wall. The idea
was for me to crouch behind the stone wall and, peering
through a three-inch hole between the stones, dart the
nilgai when it came by.

I took up my position and pressed my eye to the hole
in the wall. All I could see was a very small patch of grass.
What seemed like hours passed. My legs became cramped,

and when I shifted to a kneeling position my trousers rapidly became soaked through. The rest of me was pretty sodden anyway from the drizzle. All sorts of unpleasant thoughts went through my mind. What would happen if my field of fire was blocked by a cow passing between me and the nilgai? Suppose it went by too fast? Suppose the needle bounced back? What was the effect of phencyclidine on the nilgai? Reports on its use on such species at that time were at best not very reassuring. Suppose I missed? I would certainly lose face, I thought, among the assembled company. I remembered how, sometimes, knowing that I would have only one chance, I had overestimated the distance of an animal and pitched the trajectory of the tranquillizer syringe too high, and the missile had sailed harmlessly over the back of the animal to embed itself in the ground some yards away. All very embarrassing. One rarely gets a second chance with animals in the wild, and anyway the gun takes so long to reload that by the time a second dart is ready for firing the object of one's attention has disappeared over the horizon.

As I crouched there it occurred to me that I had been completely out of contact with the line of men for some time. I dared not stand up to see how things were progressing, in case the nilgai caught sight of me. For all I knew, everyone could have abandoned the manoeuvre and gone home without me.

Suddenly I heard the soft plopping noise of cows' feet as they walked steadily towards the gateway. They were coming! I tensed up and squinted along the barrel of my gun, which occupied most of the space in the hole. All I saw was the blurred green of the grass. Then it happened: The green turned to black, then to snow white, then to black again and back to green. A Friesian cow had walked across the other side of the hole. A moment later, the black-white, black-white flash was repeated.

I began to sweat. It seemed to take only a micro-
second for the full length of a Friesian cow to pass across
my field of fire. There were, it was said, about twenty-five
head of cattle. Somewhere among the twenty-five was the
nilgai. Perhaps it had already passed through in line abreast.
Or perhaps, sensing danger, it had left the herd and charged
off in an altogether different direction. I found it immensely difficult to avoid standing up for a quick look to
size up the situation.

Black-white, black-white—another cow—then suddenly there was a new colour. The hole was filled with a
grey-blue blur. What was more, the grey-blue blur stopped
still for a moment and I was looking down the barrel at
the gently heaving side of a nilgai antelope.

I pulled the trigger and with great relief heard the
phut of carbon dioxide gas as the missile shot through the
wall and slapped into the body of the target. With a grunt
and a scuffling noise as its hooves sought a firm hold in
the muddy gateway, the nilgai disappeared from view and
I stood up and looked anxiously over the wall. Disappear-
ing into the distance was the galloping antelope pursued by
a group of panting men. But I could see the red flash of
the tassel on the end of the dart syringe still attached to
its side. It had been done. Even now the sedative drug
would be working its way through the system towards the
brain. And, sure enough, the men eventually caught up
with the nilgai, now grown dopey and unco-ordinated.
The day ended triumphantly. The animal was recaptured,
and it recovered uneventfully from its dose of phencyclidine.

Mr. Bloom, the director, was delighted, and he invited
me to accompany him back to Flamingo Park. Would I
care to examine a giraffe with which they were having a
great deal of trouble? Instead of driving directly home, I
followed him over the moors and down to Flamingo Park,

and he showed me a female giraffe that was limping severely on one of her hind legs. They had been treating her for many months to no avail, and it was getting to the point that euthanasia had to be considered. I examined the troublesome leg. The knee joint was greatly enlarged and had a crunchy kind of feeling when I squeezed it. Because of the pain in the leg, Mr. Bloom had doubts as to whether she would ever be able to breed. It didn't seem as if she would be able to stand the weight of a male during the brief act of mating.

At that time I didn't have an X-ray machine powerful enough to penetrate a mass of bone as thick as this injured joint, but I decided to see if the X-rays from my portable set could produce at least some information by providing a picture of the silhouette of the kneecap. I took the picture, and the X-rays did show up well the area where the soft tissue covered the outline of the patella. Looking carefully at the X-ray plate I could see a small dent in the front surface of the kneecap, which surely must represent the end of a fracture. I felt certain that the problem was one of the after-effects of a fractured knee, caused perhaps by a blow or kick from the female's mate, so I treated the giraffe by injecting drugs in long acting gel form deep into the joint cavity of the knee. I asked to be kept informed of the animal's progress and then left for home.

Although she was never to lose the somewhat enlarged and knobbly knee, the giraffe did become sound again on the affected leg and walked freely without pain. So the second case that I attended to for Mr. Bloom also had a successful termination, and the big bonus was when, a couple of years later, the giraffe was safely delivered of a healthy youngster.

Now that I was visiting Flamingo Park purely out of personal interest in the young pumas, I took the opportunity to call in at Mr. Bloom's office to say hello as a matter of courtesy. While I was there a slight, rather diffident-looking man in an old mac and a pair of sandals walked in. This was Pentland Hick, the owner of Flamingo Park and a group of other zoos, exhibition halls, and leisure centres throughout Great Britain. A brilliant entrepreneur and business innovator, he was a pioneer of the boom in new forms of commercial zoo development in Europe. He was also an expert entomologist and a financial genius whose interests ranged from the theory and practice of car parking (on bank holidays he would don a white coat and personally supervise the correct positioning of vehicles at Flamingo Park) to futuristic plans to build a vertical skyscraper zoo in the heart of a big city.

After I had been introduced to him, Hick looked me over. "I believe you did some good work for us with the nilgai and the giraffe," he said. "What do you think of our zoo?"

I looked at the rather unimpressive figure. So this was the renowned Pentland Hick, I thought, pleased at his reference to the cases I had treated.

Before I could answer, he spoke again. "Perhaps you could be of some help to us. We could do with a veterinary officer here. Do you know anything about whales and dolphins?"

"I'm afraid not," I replied, "but I'm willing to learn."

Hick certainly didn't waste any words in getting to the point. "OK," he said. "Think about it when you go home, and send me your written proposals as to how veterinary supervision of my zoo group could be efficiently set up. Oh, and by the way, there's a conference the day after tomorrow in San Francisco on dolphin and whale medicine. Why don't you go over there? Send me the bill." With that he nodded, muttered his good-byes, and disappeared out of the door.

I was amazed. "Is he serious?" I asked Mr. Bloom. "Does he really want me to go off at the drop of a hat?"

"That's Pentland Hick," replied the director. "If he says it he means it. He never asks twice. You go. That's my advice."

As I was saying good-bye to Mr. Bloom, Pentland Hick popped his head round the door again. "Just one thing I forgot to say," he said. "While you're out there, better go and look at Sea World and all the other American marinelands, and don't forget the San Diego Zoo and the American Navy research centre in California." He disappeared again.

I went out into the zoo to find Shelagh, who was naturally at the puma cage being made a terrible fuss over by Morecambe and Wise. The keeper had let her go in to them, and they were sitting at her feet, gazing affectionately up into her face and whistling away for all they were worth. I was relieved to find that their new quarters were spacious, airy, and sunlit, and that they had warm, draught-free sleeping boxes and a long grassy paddock run.

Shelagh also gave their accommodations her seal of approval, and she was as delighted and astonished as I when I told her how a thirty-second conversation with Hick had resulted in an opportunity to visit the United States for the first time in my life. As soon as we got back home, I rang British Airways and booked a seat to San Francisco and then began work on a series of proposals for establishing the post of Group Veterinary Officer in control of animal health at Pentland Hick's zoos. I was writing myself into the job of a lifetime.

That trip to America was to be the first of many visits in which I learned the whole business of catching, caring for, transporting, and dealing with the medical problems of aquatic mammals. My proposals for supervising the health care at Hick's zoos were accepted, and Hick saw to it that I had a continuing post-graduate education in every aspect of zoo management. In the years that followed he would send me to survey sites for new zoos and on buying trips to animal dealers and collections in Holland, Germany, and Scandinavia. He would let me wrestle with lawyers and architects and salesmen, involving me in the planning and building and the day-to-day maintenance problems of his zoos. I would go off to scour the resorts of southern England for sites suitable for the installation of a dolphinarium or a "Devil's Zoo" collection of dangerous and bizarre creatures; I would negotiate with Madame Tussaud's Waxworks in London a new concept of animal exhibition, where models and live animals would be combined and the public could experience life in the jungle from early morning to late at night, passing from arctic conditions to tropical rain forests all in the space of half an hour.

Although some of my expeditions were failures and some of the business deals did not bear fruit, Hick never ceased to encourage me. "If only one in ten of our ideas comes to pass," he used to say, "that will be sufficient."

In brief, my meeting with Pentland Hick changed my life, resulting in an immense broadening of the scope of my experience and of my thinking about zoos and zoo animals. From then on I never really looked back. Fate moves in odd ways, but I never imagined that it would manifest itself in two little cubs named Morecambe and Wise.

4 Going Ape

ONE OF THE FIRST THINGS I did as the new vet at Flamingo
Park Zoo was to arrange for a mate-swap. Adam, the
orang-utan at Belle Vue, had never produced any offspring
during his years in Manchester, and the blame was put on
him since we could find nothing wrong with any of his
wives. Similarly Harold, the male orang at Flamingo Park
Zoo, had not been blessed with heirs. We decided to swap
Adam for Harold to see if an exchange of mates would
remedy the situation. By this time I had a dart-gun, of
course, and I decided to dart Adam, drive him over to
Flamingo Park, do the same to Harold, and carry him back
to Manchester. The orangs could sit beside me in my car.

On the day of the exchange I loaded a couple of
syringes with phencyclidine and carefully greased the
needle points with penicillin cream to deal with any germs
that might be lurking on the animals' dusty skin. Adam
was soon lightly anaesthetized. We carried him to my car
and sat him on the front seat; the safety belt kept him
nicely in position. I set off, with Adam sitting stupefied
next to me. He was in a sort of twilight world and with
any luck would not start coming round for a couple of
hours, long enough for me to make Flamingo Park—just.

To be on the safe side I put a loaded syringe containing another dose of phencyclidine on the shelf below the dashboard. This is a wise precaution. I have once or twice managed to stick an injection into the ham muscle of an ape while bowling along the motorway and holding the wheel with one hand. Such irresponsible driving cannot be recommended, but it becomes essential when the anthropoid co-driver rouses quicker than anticipated and reaches for the gearshift as a support or tries to pick his ear with the directional signal.

I reached Flamingo Park uneventfully with Adam, who was still too dreamy when we put him into the orang house with his two new wives to appreciate the touching way they brought presents of lettuce to their lord and master. With Adam safely installed, I darted Harold and had him carried to my car and without further delay set off back to Manchester.

It was a hot day, and Harold turned out to be a trifle flatulent. It became very necessary to wind down the windows. The orang sat comfortably behind the safety belt in the passenger seat on my left, his legs dangling over the edge of the seat and his arms in his lap. By the time I reached Leeds it was obvious that Harold's liver was a much more efficient destroyer of phencyclidine than Adam's and that the drug was rapidly being broken down by his system. The first signs were when Harold slowly stuck his arm out of the window and began to clench and unclench his leathery hand in the typical manner of an ape under light phencyclidine anaesthesia. A glance told me that I would have to top him up with a bit more dope in order to reach Manchester, and I decided to stop and attend to him as soon as I had cleared the busy traffic of Leeds city centre.

Harold fidgeted slightly in his seat and began slowly

to lick his lips. His other hand was now creeping slowly, ever so slowly, around the base of the gearshift. Still barely conscious of what he was doing, Harold drooled while the strong, thick fingers of his right hand unpicked a piece of plastic trim with a loud *crack*. The index finger of the hand, moving as if with a mind of its own, entered the hole it had made and gained purchase on a bigger piece of plastic. *Crack!* At this rate I would be driving on a naked chassis by the time I reached Huddersfield. There were red traffic lights ahead. As soon as I got through them I would pull up and give him the knock-out drops.

I stopped at the lights in the middle of the three lanes of traffic. On our left waited a paper boy on a bicycle, his canvas bag of newspapers slung over his shoulder. He was too busy watching for the green light to notice the fat, red-haired drunk sitting in a car by his elbow. The lights changed and I let out the clutch, my eye fixed on a place a couple of hundred yards ahead where I might park briefly. Suddenly there was a piercing yell.

I looked in my mirror. Nothing to see.

"Ooooow! He-e-e-y!"

There was the cry again, somewhere to my left and behind me. I slowed down and looked over Harold's head. Stuck like a fly to the outside of my car was the paper boy. His bicycle was lying some yards behind in the middle of the road. But what was the adhesive that made him cling so closely to the vehicle's side? Then I saw that Harold's wandering left hand had come across the boy's canvas bag when we were stopped at the lights. As soon as we moved off the hand had tightened powerfully by reflex action round the canvas sling of the bag, and the lad had been dragged off his bike like a stone from a catapult.

I stopped and went round to release Harold's catch.

Fortunately the boy was not injured. I retrieved his bicycle, introduced him to the drowsing ape, and let him hold my bottle while I prepared more dope. The lad soon recovered his wits, and I rather fancy that being unhorsed by an orang-utan made his day. I still wonder whether anyone believed him when he went home and related how, like something out of a crazy gangster film, a car had pulled up alongside him in the middle of Leeds and a fat, ugly orang-utan had tried to kidnap him. But I'm certain that he would have been as delighted as I was to learn that the orang swap resulted in the birth of babies at both zoos the following year.

As my practice slowly expanded, I became accustomed to driving up to 700 miles a day within Britain. On numerous occasions I would set off early in the morning, drive up to a safari park in Scotland to see a sick dolphin, and then immediately turn round and drive the whole length of England down to Windsor to attend to an ailing rhinoceros. Having dealt with that I would then set off north again and drive the 250 miles to my home, calling in at Belle Vue on the way to do the weekly report on the animals in quarantine and attend to any other outstanding cases. Luckily, and strangely enough, I cannot ever recall an occasion when two equally urgent emergency cases occurred simultaneously at opposite ends of the country or in two widely separated points in Europe. Providence seems to have looked kindly upon my exotic animals. Although two, three, or even four emergencies in different zoos throughout my practice might blow up almost at the same time, it has always been possible by dint of furious driving and careful co-ordination of airline timetables to get to each patient within the same day.

The animals, therefore, may not have suffered unduly, but I have had (quite willingly) to pay some penalties in loss of sleep or spent uncomfortable nights trying to catch some rest curled up in my car, parked by the roadside. Frequent assaults have been made on my otherwise iron digestive system by a succession of missed meals and hurriedly ingested meat pies, and I have acquired a remarkably high turnover rate in vehicles, a persistent tendency to cancellation of social engagements, and a succession of speeding fines from the unsympathetic judiciary which once culminated in a six months' driving ban.

The long journeys which were necessary between zoos in Britain meant that I was out in all weather conditions at all times of the day, and on a winter day several months after the Harold-Adam exchange I found myself having to drive down to the London dolphinarium on a particularly miserable foggy day to see a sick dolphin. After treating the dolphin, I decided to stay in London overnight and travel north in the morning. The weather was getting worse, and a freezing fog had clamped down over London. Conditions on the M.1 freeway that runs to the north of England would be atrocious.

Just then the telephone in the dolphinarium rang. It was Ray Legge, the director of Belle Vue, and he was in big trouble with his gorillas.

"What seems to be the matter, Ray?" I asked.

"It's Suzy," he replied. "She's flat out, cold and blue."

"What do you think happened?" I asked.

"It's as cold as hell up here, freezing fog, terrible night, and to cap it all the underfloor heating has conked out. Must have been like that for several hours. How soon can you get up?"

"I'll set off straight away," I replied. "The way the weather is I may not get back till two in the morning, but I'll be up as fast as I can. In the meantime see if you can warm her up and get some strong sweet tea into her."

I set off for the north. It took me an hour and a half

just to reach the freeway. Once there, conditions were
even worse. The road surface was glazed with black ice,
and white clouds of dense fog obliterated sight of everything except the lane markers. It was like driving in all-
enveloping cotton wool. I calculated that if it was like this
all the way up to Manchester and I was kept down to a
constant five miles an hour it would take me two days to
reach the gorilla.

I edged my way cautiously onwards. Suddenly there
was a short, sharp explosion. Something, possibly a stone
thrown up by a vehicle ahead of me, had hit the glass like
a bullet and my windscreen had become an opaque network of fissures that veiled even the fog from my eyes. I
punched a hole in the glass with my clenched fist. Little
chunks of glass began to dislodge themselves from the
rough edge of the hole. I was forced to pluck out insecure
splinters as I drove along, making the hole bigger and
bigger.

Eventually all the remaining pieces of windscreen fell
away, leaving me completely exposed to the elements. It
was bitterly cold. Fog swirled into the car, chilling me to
the marrow. The car heater seemed to have given up the
ghost. The fog thinned a little and I was able to increase
speed slightly, but the faster I drove the colder I became.
I was literally seizing up. It became increasingly difficult
to grasp the gearshift. Steering and concentration on the
foggy road ahead became increasingly difficult. At last,
just as my morale was beginning to sink to a very low ebb,
I glimpsed through the murk a sign indicating a service
station one mile ahead. Somehow I limped into it and
managed to drag myself into the cafeteria to consume great
draughts of hot tea.

Revived, I returned to the car and put on every garment I could find. Three extra shirts, one jacket squeezed

on top of another, two more old shirts wrapped round each thigh. I crammed newspapers down my trousers and under my sweater, and over all I wore an old raincoat and finally my duffel coat. Then I set off again, out along the freeway with the fog getting icier as the night wore on.

I had hardly travelled two miles before my defences had been penetrated. The cold got in again and I began once more to chill rapidly. I tried bouncing in my seat, throwing my body to left and right as I clung to the wheel, beating a tattoo with my feet, but it was to no avail. The cold became sheer agony and despair tightened its grip upon me. For the first time in my career I was going to have to ring and say I couldn't do the job. Suzy would have to get along without me. But to telephone, I would have to get to the next service station twenty miles farther on.

On and on I crawled, and eventually, almost dizzy with numbness, I reached the station and pulled in. More hot drinks and a spell in the warmth of the cafeteria revived me once again, and the despair faded away as warmth returned to my limbs. I decided to try to make it just from one service station to another, to forget about my ultimate goal and just concentrate upon surviving one lap at a time. There were five more stations to go. At least in the filthy conditions no one else seemed to be moving on the road. Truck drivers and police in the cafeterias I stopped at shook their heads when they saw me preparing to leave again.

"Must be a ruddy fool driving in conditions like this," I heard one say as I left, readjusting my newspaper packing and straining to close my duffel coat as it bulged over the padded frame beneath.

"Some mothers do 'ave 'em," another replied.

Tacking from one service station to the next, I pro-

gressed along the freeway system. Gradually the fog
thinned and I was able to pick up a little more speed, although the temperature remained well below zero. Eventually, at nearly four o'clock in the morning, I pulled into
the zoo gardens in Manchester and drove straight to the
great ape house.

Ray Legge was waiting for me. He looked tired and
worried. "Thank God you've arrived," he said. "Come and
look at Suzy. I haven't been able to do much for her.
Jo-Jo won't let me get into their sleeping quarters, and I
can't split him off. What's more, I think he's the cause of
the trouble."

I looked into the gorilla cage. Suzy was lying motionless on the floor while Jo-Jo sat snugly—and smugly—
in a large pile of wood wool in his sleeping recess. He
looked down at me and adjusted the bedding around his
toes. There wasn't even a scrap of wood wool in the sleeping recess that was normally used by Suzy, nor was there
any lying on the floor. It was fairly obvious what had
happened, for it was still cold in the great ape house even
though the director had set up hot air blowers as soon as
he had found the collapsed gorilla. With the underfloor
heating out of action on such a bitterly cold night, Jo-Jo
had decided to look after Number One. I can imagine him
assiduously collecting every scrap of bedding for himself
and then driving off Suzy when she tried to make up a
double bed.

I had seen this greedy type of behaviour on the part of
male orangs and gorillas on previous occasions, not necessarily related to cold weather. Like human males, great
apes sometimes treat their womenfolk very badly: They
will jealously hoard food that they do not possibly want
to eat, and they will sometimes keep driving their mates
away from water pots long after they themselves have had

a surfeit of drink. In the gorilla house at Belle Vue there are two large stainless-steel feeding trays which pass through slots in the wall, one for each gorilla. When both are filled with fruit and vegetables I have seen Jo-Jo dashing greedily from one tray to the other, trying to monopolize both lots of food. He will eat at one tray until he sees Suzy trying to take a nibble at the other, when he will petulantly charge over to Suzy's tray, whereupon Suzy moves to the now vacated tray and the whole rigmarole is repeated.

Now it looked as if Suzy, suffering from hypothermia, was simply chilling away to death. Whether Jo-Jo liked it or not, I was going to examine her, and to do that Jo-Jo would have to be rendered unconscious. Treating Suzy was going to be difficult enough without having three hundred pounds of muscle-bound male gorilla complicating matters.

Jo-Jo seemed to know what I was thinking, for he left his sleeping recess, clambered down, and ambled across to the armoured window that separated us from him. He looked up at me sagely and projected a round high-speed blob of saliva which popped against the glass right between my eyes, as it were.

For underhand spitting Jo-Jo wins the prize. What he lacks in accuracy he makes up for in sneakiness. Jo-Jo's centrally heated, stainless-steel-fitted quarters have heavy metal doors, and it is through a small spyhole in one of these doors that I poke my dart-gun when trying to anaesthetize him. These occasions come fairly regularly, since all medical examinations mean dartings; you cannot handle a three-hundred-pound male gorilla any other way. So Jo-Jo knows that the spyhole in the door is something of a nuisance.

The procedure usually goes like this. First I put my

eye to the hole to see where Jo-Jo is. I then load the dart-gun while Jo-Jo looks back through the hole at me. I can just see one dark shining eye. I return to the hole to see where Jo-Jo is positioned and *wham!* A ball of spittle zips through the hole and hits me in the eye. Having wiped my face I poke the gun through the hole and squint down the barrel. There is just enough room for me to see what I am aiming at. No gorilla: Jo-Jo is crouching close to the door below my line of sight and suddenly grabs the metal gun barrel. He cannot haul the whole weapon through the small hole, but he has a good try. His next move is to spike my gun before I can get a bead on him. He pops up, opens his mouth, and spits long and hard up the barrel of my gun. I withdraw the weapon for on-the-spot de-spitting and Jo-Jo moves back to the hole. As I busy myself cleaning the barrel I feel a blob of warm, sticky saliva hit the back of my neck. First rounds always go to Jo-Jo.

So here I was once again having to deal with my old friend and adversary. I loaded the dart-gun with tran-quillizer, we played the inevitable "spit up the barrel" game, but within a few minutes the great fellow was dreaming peacefully on his back beside Suzy, his arms crossed on his bulging paunch like a drunken Sumo wrestler.

We opened the metal door and entered the gorillas' quarters. Suzy was lying as if she too had been tranquillized and the colour of her gums was pale and bluish. I anxiously felt her scalp, fingers, toes. They were all chilled. I took her pulse and listened to her heart through my stethoscope. The circulation was weak, the respiration was depressed, and there were faint but ominous liquid bubbling sounds in the lower edges of both lungs.

While Ray Legge brought portable heaters into the den itself, I prepared injections to stimulate the circulation and to protect against pneumonia and administered them into Suzy's forearm vein for quickest effect. She wasn't completely unconscious, and still had a swallowing reflex, so I decided to try to give some central liquid energy. Very carefully, I spooned a syrupy mixture of sugar and water at blood heat between her lips. She managed to swallow it, with Ray Legge propping her up into a sitting position so that we minimized the chances of any of the liquid going down the wrong way and either drowning the animal or starting up the so-called aspiration pneumonia so frequently seen where weak, unconscious, or very old animals or humans are too rapidly force-fed when lying in unnatural positions.

When half a pint of the warm, nourishing liquid had disappeared safely inside her, I decided to dress Suzy up. Taking off the duffel coat and some of the shirts and sweaters which had helped me to survive the trip up from London and were now warm with my body heat, we struggled to get Suzy into them, and eventually she was clad, if not elegantly, at least adequately to insulate her better against heat loss.

Ray Legge went off to fetch more hot air blowers and the entire supply of cotton wool stored in our dispensary. While he was away I began rubbing Suzy's limbs as hard as I could. I hoped this would stimulate the blood flow back to the heart and carry warmth to the deeper organs of the body, and, indeed, little by little Suzy's colour improved. She began to move her head and blink her eyes, and I felt her fingers pluck ever so gently at my jacket. I monitored her heart action. It was becoming stronger, and the pulse was not as thin and thready as it had been when I first arrived. Suzy was beginning to recover.

When Ray Legge returned we split the gorilla den

into two by winding down the metal dividing wall and made up two comfortable beds of deep cotton wool and wood wool, one on either side. I wasn't going to have Jo-Jo doing any more thieving of bedding when he recovered from my knock-out dose. While Ray Legge continued massaging poor Suzy, I pulled the slumbering Jo-Jo into bed by his legs, turning him on his side, making sure that his tongue could not fall back and choke him, and covering him with a blanket of cotton wool. Then I stood back to admire the deceptively innocent face with its closed eyes and the faintest hint of a sardonic smile on its lips.

Having got Jo-Jo settled, I went back to the director and Suzy. She was now rousing and seemed to be enjoying the vigorous rubbing of her arms and legs. From time to time she looked down at the clothes she was wearing and toyed with the buttons. She'd never before worn a stitch in her life. She was getting to the point at which I thought it would be safe to give her a drop of hard liquor. Although alcohol is bad for severely chilled patients, it does have restorative properties when the major heat loss problem has been overcome.

We made up three glasses with double shots of Scotch, lemon juice, brown sugar, grated nutmeg, and hot water—one glass for Suzy, one for Ray Legge, and the third for me. It was a warming breakfast, for the time was now a little before seven. When Suzy had finished hers, she turned the glass upside down and peered into it, as if wanting the last drop to fall in her eye. This was her sign for "more of the same if you please, and look sharp about it before I scrunch up the glass." After another generous slug of the mixture, Suzy was glowing with warmth, superbly good-natured, but rapidly becoming more vigorous. Taking an arm and a leg each, we put her to bed. Just before tucking her in I took back my duffel coat and sweater but decided to leave a couple of shirts on her. The two layers of air trapped beneath them would insulate her nicely until the mechanics came to mend the central heating in a couple of hours. Wearily we locked the cage, put out the lights, and went home.

Suzy wore my shirts very proudly for the next few weeks. She recovered completely and was again reunited with her mate, but her first set of clothes seemed to have driven a new determination into her soul. She was definitely not going to part with them. Whenever Jo-Jo came strutting up in his overbearing way with an eye to ripping off and purloining the garments, he found that a touch of fashion had made the worm turn, for she would set upon him, arms flailing, teeth bared, and voice bawling in a tone that unmistakably signified "over my dead body!" Jo-Jo got the message and tried, I thought, to convey the impression that he could not care less for such feminine vanities. Nevertheless, when eventually the shirts literally fell to pieces and Suzy had to abandon her short-lived finery, Jo-Jo could sometimes be seen quietly picking up the shreds and pieces, sneaking back to the sleeping recess, and there, back turned towards onlookers, vainly trying to get them to fit together in one piece around his bulging torso.

5 Flamingo Park

Now THAT I was a full-time zoo vet, I wanted very much to get a taste of the day-to-day running of an animal collection. The vet working in a zoo usually sees only one side of the animal-keeping business: He will drop in, examine a case, prescribe treatment, and disappear again, talking only with the director and the head keeper and having little time to study the actual running of what is, after all, a kind of farm for exotic species. Vets in domestic large-animal practice know how to milk cows, ride horses, and discuss knowledgeably with the farmers the state of the hay harvest or the market price for wool; it's an integral part of their professionalism. I saw no reason why it should be otherwise for a vet in a zoo.

By chance it was again Pentland Hick who gave me the opportunity. Only a few months after my first meeting with him a vacancy for a curator occurred at Flamingo Park, and to my delight he asked me if I would like to fill it for a while. I would double up as Group Veterinary Officer and live for most of the week at the park in a trailer at the bottom of the zoo.

I accepted with alacrity, although I made it clear that at the end of something between six and twelve months

I would want to return to Rochdale to continue my exotic animal consultancy. (As things turned out, I stayed at Flamingo Park for a year and a half after moving up to the post of assistant director.) Hick agreed that while at the park I could travel as freely as I wished to treat cases of my other clients. Shelagh wasn't too keen on the idea of my spending five or six days a week away from home, but she saw how badly I wanted to do it and understood the value of the experience. For my girls, Stephanie and Lindsey, the sweetener would be having the trailer for weekend visits when the weather was good. Up till that time I had driven over to see my patients at Flamingo Park, doing the round trip of 200 miles—over the rugged Pennine hills, down through the industrial city of Leeds, across the lush countryside surrounding the ancient walled city of York, through the bottlenecks of the brewing centre of Tadcaster and the sleepy market town of Malton —sometimes twice and, on one hectic occasion, when unrelated emergencies came in rapid succession, three times a day. It was going to be both relaxing and interesting actually living on the job.

I certainly jumped in at the deep end, and although I was a medical man accustomed to giving opinions and expecting my advice to be respected and heeded (I had been practicing for over eleven years by this time), the zoo director made it plain from the very first that I would have to carry the can for my staff of twenty-one keepers and work in just the same way as any other curator.

Curators are theoretically the custodians of an animal collection. Some zoos have several of them: one in charge of mammals, another of birds, another of reptiles, and so forth. At Flamingo Park there was just one, responsible to the zoo director for the day-to-day maintenance and display of the exhibits and with a hierarchy of head keeper, senior keepers, keepers in charge of particular sections, assistant keepers, and trainees under him.

Inevitably the obvious responsibilities of the curator for purely animal welfare matters extend into a whole spectrum of related affairs which involve other non-zoological departments: food supply, staffing, hygiene, the needs and desires of the paying public, and the commercial strategy of the board of directors. If an animal is ill and "off show," its unavailability may affect bookings for, say, the Dolphinarium, the times of shows, the need for overtime, and, as a further extension, the receipts at the main gates, the numbers of coach parties to be prepared for by catering, and the weekly advertising tactics. The curator has to wrestle with the farm manager over grazing and fodder supplies, cater to the whims of the publicity department, and coax the repairs to animal houses and the building of transporting crates out of the engineer in competition with similar demands from the manager of the trailer park or the head gardener.

And the compass of the curator's work at Flamingo Park went further still, a fact of which I was blithely unaware when I accepted Hick's offer. It was a baptism in ice-cold water. I had to struggle very hard to suppress my resentment when, on the first morning after I took up the position, the zoo director called me into his office and ticked me off for a host of oversights of which I was completely unaware. No list of instructions, no standing orders, not even an oral briefing had gone with the job, but there he sat behind his desk with me standing before him, feeling like a schoolboy up before the Head for stealing apples.

He wanted to know why somebody had left a small window in the monkey house open all night; didn't I know it was my job to make a final check to make sure that everything was secure? A keeper had been seen spending an unusually large quantity of verdigris-covered pennies in the cafeteria. Hadn't I better look into it? He might have been fishing in the alligator pool, which, as in most reptile houses, takes its toll of small coins from the public, who either try to stimulate the torpid beasts with these handy missiles or look on the pool as a potential wishing well. Another thing: The Easter crowds would soon be here. Had I checked to see that the toilets were in good working condition? Yes, the toilet block was under my control as well, as was first-aid. If I were wise I would keep an eye on the time clock system, too. There'd been some fiddles recently, and while I was about it, make sure that the lads didn't go overboard in claiming overtime. There had been evidence of overfeeding and wastage of expensive fruit in the monkey house. And so on. Long before the end of the rather acerbic interview it had dawned on me that my duties embraced virtually every activity in the park except handling the cash, feeding the human visitors, and dealing with the vagaries of the temperamental park sewage disposal plant.

And so they did. For instance, because emergency firearms and, of course, the dart-guns were in my care, it seemed logical to have me also look after the pistols and blank cartridges of the Cowboy City sideshow down in the fun-fair. The trouble was, having once inherited their weapons, I found myself saddled with all their other problems as well, such as supplying keepers as stand-ins on busy afternoons when the "redskins" in their group didn't turn up for work and showing the "marshal" how to harness up his stagecoach team, a task he never properly mastered.

I was also responsible for such things as nipping in the bud the first signs of moral turpitude among the male and female members of my staff who lived on the grounds and keeping the local Hunt from riding across our land. I was also in charge of cooling things diplomatically when, as regularly happened, the peacocks got into the tiny country church that abutted the zoo and interrupted the vicar's sermons with their peculiarly piercing, eerie cries. "By the way," said the director the first time the peacocks escaped, "try to wait until there's a hymn in progress before you grab 'em. It doesn't sound so bad. You *are* Church of England, I presume?"

At times I wondered if I had made the right decision. But I hung on and was rewarded. There was much to be learned, for instance, in watching Violet, the lady in charge of the animal kitchen. She may have had no theoretical nutritional knowledge, but her hygiene and practical precision were impeccable, and she consistently created a galaxy of appetizing and aesthetically pleasing diets for every one of the creatures in the zoo, working from charts of each species' essential requirements that I had prepared. There was the opportunity to put into practice some of my ideas about making the pens, paddocks, and houses in which animals were kept more hospitable and thus more likely to encourage breeding. I was present at more zoo animal births than I had ever witnessed before. My contacts with other zoos throughout the world expanded, and I began to learn more of the commercial aspects of animal buying and selling. And, of course, the whole was leavened by the regular trickle of veterinary work.

However, during the summer I treated more small boys than animals, for cuts, bloody noses, and abrasions— and some of the human emergencies were more serious than that.

One of the first things I had to deal with after moving into Flamingo Park was a rattlesnake which was growing thinner and thinner because of so-called maladaptation. This is an extremely common condition in snakes, particularly newly arrived ones, which are physically and psychologically distressed by changes in habitat, temperature, and humidity and simply stop eating in their new environment and—if left alone—will starve themselves to death. It then becomes necessary to force-feed the snake. One of my preferred methods is to pass a small plastic stomach tube down the throat of the reptile and then pump in a thick liquid puree of raw liver, egg, vitamin powder, and water. The reptile keeper holds the snake firmly with both hands just behind the head, while I pass the tube—a simple operation.

The Flamingo Park rattler had only been with us a few weeks, and the vivarium in which we put it seemed satisfactory to me in every respect. I decided that the snake must have been upset by the long trip from Miami; it had travelled tied in a muslin bag which had been put in a cardboard box together with half a dozen other snakes, similarly packaged. In time, I hoped it would settle down and begin to eat. Until then it would be necessary to give thrice weekly force-feeds.

After helping with a couple of doses via the stomach tube, the reptile keeper assured me that he would be quite capable of doing the force-feeding by himself in the future. Foolishly, I agreed. A few days later, when filling up the rattlesnake again, the keeper was bitten deeply on the hand and I was summoned.

The danger in force-feeding snakes without an assistant occurs at one brief but crucial point. After the snake has been trapped by an L- or Y-shaped rod, the catcher then bends down and grasps the reptile firmly behind the head with the right hand. Casting aside the rod, he lifts up the snake and prepares to pass the stomach tube. To do this a right-handed man will want to transfer the snake into his left hand so that he can guide the tube carefully between the teeth, through the pharynx, and, avoiding the windpipe, down the gullet into the stomach. It is this transfer of the snake from the right to the left hand which produces a split second of jeopardy. Unless one takes the greatest care to maintain a constant grip with the thumb and forefinger of both hands at all times during the transfer, there occurs a moment when neither is fully in control of the lethal mouth parts. It needs only that trice for the reptile's fangs to be plunged into the man's flesh.

I dashed into the tropical house and saw the reptile keeper sitting, white and shocked, staring at the two small brown holes in the base of his thumb. Already his hand was beginning to puff up, and I noticed large beads of sweat growing on his forehead. Malton, the nearest town, had only a small cottage hospital. I sent someone to telephone them and warn them that a snake-bite victim was on the way. I felt miserably responsible for the whole affair as I ran to get my car. It would be quicker to take him in than to wait for an ambulance to arrive. I'd learned a valuable lesson: here we were keeping venomous snakes but there wasn't a drop of anti-venom serum on the premises or within a hundred miles. It seems a limp thing to say that we had never thought of it, but that was the wretched truth, and even today many zoos and the vast majority of venomous snake owners still do not make arrangements for either themselves or their local hospital to store supplies of the specific antidotes for snake bite.

When I got the reptile keeper into the front seat of my car, his perspiring white face had taken on a new shade of green. He was collapsing. Death from shock sometimes occurs in such circumstances. I had no intention of applying a tight tourniquet above the wound or of slashing deeply into the fang marks with a knife and sucking out the blood and venom, the standard procedures described in yarns of intrepid jungle explorers; such measures can produce far more serious effects than the venom itself. Instead, I decided to do something that was rare indeed for me—give a human an injection.

I hadn't time to think of the implications for me if anything went wrong. I whipped open the trunk of my car, fumbled for an unopened bottle of cortico-steroid, filled a 1-cc disposable syringe, and went back to the sick man. Tearing open a hole in his shirt sleeve, I plunged the needle into his upper arm. The cortico-steroid, a preparation I carried for treating arthritic monkeys and giraffes, would, I hoped, fend off the serious effects of shock until I got him to the hospital. Then, while I drove, I reached Belle Vue over my radio telephone and asked them to send their supplies of anti-rattlesnake serum under police escort over to Yorkshire.

By the time I arrived at the little cottage hospital the reptile keeper was almost unconscious, and his hand, now was swollen to four times its size, was mottled black and ugly red. It was the hospital's first case of rattlesnake bite, but once he was there the condition of the keeper began to level out, and within an hour, sirens screaming, a police car drew up bearing the doses of rattlesnake anti-venom. The human body often doesn't take kindly to being given what amounts to a mini-transfusion from a completely unrelated species, the horse, and our patient turned out to be highly sensitive to the serum. He recovered quickly from the effects of the snake bite but spent three weeks in hospital overcoming the unpleasant effects produced on his system by the curative injections of serum.

After this episode I wondered what would happen if I were bitten by one of the venomous snakes I treat. A short time before, and I can pinpoint the exact day precisely, I had myself become very definitely allergic to the protein molecules of the horse family. For years I had treated the surgical problems of horses, donkeys, and increasingly more exotic equines such as the zebra, onager, and wild ass, in the process naturally coming into intimate contact with their body fluids. I had never had the slightest reaction until one night Shelagh had asked me to look at a decrepit old horse. As secretary of the Horses and Ponies Protection Association, an organization dedicated to the rescue of neglected, unwanted, and cruelly treated horses and donkeys, she had heard of a racehorse that hadn't come up to scratch and had been literally put on the scrap heap. (That was where it was found, trying to keep alive by browsing on the weeds and drinking from the rainwater trapped in the rusting metal of old car bodies.) She arranged for this pitiful creature to come and spend a period of recuperation and rehabilitation in our acre of market garden where she could keep an eye on it, and where Henry, my pet goat, a drinker of beer and consumer of vast quantities of chicken vindaloo curry, would give him companionship.

Shortly after its arrival I found the horse to be heavily parasitized by blood-sucking bowel worms and decided to give it a stiff dose of anti-worm medicine via a stomach tube. One of the reasons why I've never really enjoyed using stomach tubes on members of the horse family is that sometimes the procedure makes their noses bleed, for to get down into the gullet one starts off not as might be expected through the mouth, but up the nostrils, over the soft palate, and down into the oesophagus. Sure enough, on this occasion, once the stomach tube was safely and painlessly in position, the nose began to bleed and a few drops of blood fell on my face. Within seconds I couldn't see a thing. My cyelids puffed up like small balloons, I streamed with tears, my face swelled until I felt the skin would split, and everything from my neck upwards began to itch intolerably. When I walked back into the house, Shelagh had the fright of her life; I was unrecognizable. By some strange quirk of fate I had become unaccountably allergic to protein of equine origin.

In the end, the racehorse ended up in better shape than its doctor, for in the days that followed the phenomenon was repeated with monotonous regularity. Blood on my hands, a fleck of saliva getting into my eye, or the minutest trace of horse dander (the greasy dust or dandruff of a horse's skin) up my nose or on a tiny abrasion, and I was within a few moments transformed to a pitiably squinting, sneezing, scratching, red-faced object.

I had some success with preventive doses of antihistamine pills, but they weren't the complete answer, since they made me sleepy and not quick enough in action. Luckily over the years I seem to have improved immensely, becoming, I think, naturally desensitized to equine protein simply by having re-exposed myself to the stuff time and time again until the point has been reached at which my body's allergic defence reactions have settled down and stopped making so much fuss whenever a horsy particle or two comes in contact with my cells. However, this took a long time, and while I was at Flamingo Park my allergy was in full bloom. Indeed, it was there that one of the most severe manifestations of my horse allergy occurred.

A zebra mare was in trouble giving birth. She was a wise and relatively quiet creature and permitted me, having scrubbed up and covered my arm with a lubricant antiseptic jelly, to feel inside the birth canal and onwards into the womb to ascertain the cause of the trouble without giving her any form of dope. There are obvious advantages to keeping a mother in labour of this sort fully conscious. Having corrected any faults in the position of the young baby about to be born, there is nothing like the powerful, deep, and central voluntary pushing of the mother to help the youngster on its way. It certainly beats pulling. The trouble is that sedatives diminish and anaesthetics eliminate the mother's ability to push.

Feeling gently inside the zebra, I found that an apparently live, normal-sized foal was firmly jammed in the classical breech position. With its buttocks pointed into the vagina and its hind legs towards the chest, the little fellow was hopelessly wedged in the mother's bony pelvis so that natural birth was out of the question. To right matters I would first have to push it back where it came from. This meant using both arms, but nature has a wonderful way just before birth of relaxing and slackening all the tissues around the birth canal, and in an animal the size of a zebra there would be ample room for them.

My plan was to use my left hand to push the butt of the baby zebra firmly forward towards the interior of the womb. My right hand could then slip into the space left and fish around for the hind legs. If I could get a finger round the hock joint of first one and then the other hind leg, I could slide my grip down to the little hooves and then pull them so that both legs pointed backwards into the vagina. From then on the going would be easy and the foal would be born in the fairly normal hind-feet-first position.

As soon as I began my manipulations deep inside the warmth of the straining zebra, I began to feel my horse allergy getting under way. Immersed as they were in the natural placental liquids, my arms began to itch and puff up at an incredible rate. As I struggled to hook my right index finger round the squirming limb of the foal it felt just as if someone were pumping my arm up with air like a tyre. My fingers began to bloat and become difficult to bend. I could feel the ring of the open cervix, the entrance to the womb, squeezing round my forearms. As each minute passed I had less and less room in which to work, for I was continuing to expand to fill the space available! Working with arms at full stretch and bending only at the wrists and fingers becomes rapidly very tiring. In such cases I was accustomed to pulling out for a rest from time to time, but when I tried this I found that it was going to be an exceptionally tight squeeze. I was still swelling, and I became frightened that if I came out I might not be able to get back in again.

I decided to rest my hands by pushing farther forward in front of the foal's hind legs and jamming myself even more tightly up against the rear end of the mother. If I could find just a little room somewhere in the womb to let my hands hang and regain some of their use I could perhaps carry on and finish the job. I sweated as I strained to find a haven beside the soft belly of the foal where my aching and barely controllable digits could rest a while. A complicating factor was that the pressure of the birth canal on my swollen arms was beginning to nip my nerves and add numbness to the tribulations of my extremities.

After thirty seconds or so of inactivity bathed in the liquid warmth my hands revived a little and I felt able to seek frantically around once again for the elusive hock joints. Got 'em! I suddenly felt the familiar bowstring of an Achilles tendon at the zebra's equivalent of the human heel. More probing quickly revealed the opposite member. Giving a desperate heave, with my fingers now about as useful as a bunch of frankfurters, I dragged the two little limbs, which kicked and struggled against me quite lustily, over the rim of the pelvic bone and safely into the vagina. Slowly and painfully I withdrew my bloated arms and gave instructions for the head keeper to attach a pair of sterilized calving ropes to the little fetlock joints and assist the mother in delivering the foal by pulling steadily.

I got out just in time, for a minute or two later my hands and arms were completely numb. It took a stiff dose of antihistamine and a three-hour wait before I was ready to finish off the job by going back into the womb again and dropping off a handful of protective antiseptic pellets. Understandably, the healthy little zebra colt produced by that afternoon's exertions was named Algy, short for allergy.

Of course it is occasionally necessary to give a mother an anaesthetic in order to tackle a more complicated delivery. This happened on several occasions while I was resident at Flamingo Park. And on one occasion it resulted in my performing the first Caesarean operation ever to be recorded for a zebra.

The keepers had seen afterbirth hanging from a young Chapman's zebra mare for some hours and assumed that she had foaled and that the foal was somewhere in the zebra reserve, but a careful search revealed nothing. I examined the nervous animal at a distance through binoculars. She still had the afterbirth dangling. The fact that her belly was rounded and bulging did not necessarily mean that a foal was still in there, as zebras' shapes can be very deceptive. Then I saw her stand and lift the floor of her abdomen in a long, powerful contraction. A small white object appeared outside the birth canal and then popped back in again as she stopped straining. It was the delicate little hoof of the baby zebra emerging under pressure. I decided to leave well enough alone for two hours and then reassess the situation.

Two hours later I returned to the zebra reserve. Peering through the binoculars I saw no sign of straining, although the baby had still not been born. No part of the foal was visible and the mother seemed to be duller and more tired. All was not going well, and I decided to intervene.

Because the animal could not be closely approached, I would use the long-range dart-gun. I had found that it was possible to get closer to groups of deer, antelopes, and zebras by taking vehicles into their large paddocks rather than by going in on foot, so I decided to shoot from my car. At the time I had a Citroën saloon whose adjustable suspension made riding at speed over rough ground and firing a rifle at the same time, as if from a Western stage-coach, fairly easy. A keeper drove my car towards the mother-to-be, and when we were within range I pulled the trigger. The syringe thwacked into her buttocks. She moved a few paces, flicking at it with her tail, but the missile hits so fast it produces no more pain than a smack of a hand, so the target rarely runs off in alarm.

Five minutes later the zebra was asleep on the ground and I began my internal examination. The foal was terribly tangled up and I could detect no sign of life. Although I could unravel the awkwardly bent legs, struggle as I might I could not correctly position the head, which was bent backwards deep into the womb and also twisted round on itself. The mother's natural lubricating liquids were drying up. I had no choice but to try a Caesarean operation.

Caesareans in the horse family, of which the zebra is a member, are still not common. Horses were at one time far greater risks for this type of operation than cattle or sheep, since they get peritonitis after abdominal surgery at the drop of a hat. Until the development of modern anaesthetics and antibiotics they did not have much of a chance, and even today there are unsolved problems in doing major abdominal surgery on horses. Among zoo animals, Caesareans had quite often been performed on the big cats and on primates, but never before on zebras and other exotic horses. But this time I had no option. I had to open her up.

For a large animal like this there is rarely a spotless, aseptic operating theatre at hand so we have to work literally in the field. A tractor pulled the sleeping zebra into the stable on a sledge improvised from an old door. After reinforcing the anaesthesia by numbing the belly with local anaesthetic, I cut quickly through the skin and muscle and peritoneal tissues, bringing the bulging uterus into the light of day. As usual with wild animals, there was none of the messy fat tissue which clogs up the operation site in so many obese and pampered pets. I opened the womb and the striped leg of the foal popped out. Perhaps there was still a flicker of life. I pulled, and the slim and perfect form of the baby zebra slid out onto the side of its unconscious dam.

Ignoring the mother for the moment, I quickly opened her foal's mouth and hooked the mucus out of its throat with my fingers. Then I took it by its hind fetlocks and whirled it round and round my body as fast as possible, trying to clear its breathing tubes by centrifugal force. I stopped and listened. If its heart was beating I could not detect it. I gave an injection of stimulant and dropped some liquid on the back of the tiny tongue to kick the breathing centres into action. Still nothing. Finally I tried mouth-to-mouth respiration, packing the slippery little muzzle into my mouth and blowing as hard as I could. It was no use. The foal could not respond. It was dead.

The mother still had to be saved for her next child. I scrubbed up again and went back to work stitching up the layers in the operation wound. Before closing the abdomen I left behind in the peritoneal cavity a handful of antibiotic tablets and sprayed the bowels with a chemical to stop peritonitis from sticking them together. Finally I sutured the tough skin, tearing my fingers as I gripped the large curved needles with their cutting edges. Finished. The zebra was breathing strongly. Surprisingly little blood had been lost during the operation, hardly more than a tablespoonful. I gave her a precautionary dose of antibiotics injected into her neck and watched as she came out from under the anaesthetic, snorted, righted herself, rose, and walked sedately out to the zebra reserve. I was happy to see her go, for the reserve was a much cleaner place for post-operative recovery than a dusty stable.

The zebra never looked back. She recovered superbly from the operation without the slightest hint of complications. And the following year she produced unobserved and unaided, the most charming little filly one could wish to see.

6 Man vs. Beast

AT THE END OF THE 1960s, during my stint as curator, Flamingo Park was the first of the new-style country parks in Great Britain. Combining elements of a stately home with formal gardens, fairground, and picnic and trailer sites around a nucleus of a large walk-around zoo, it was a forerunner of the safari park, which was in some senses shortly to supersede it. Flamingo Park never closed, even on Christmas Day, and the grounds were open to the public virtually round the clock. Along with its open plan necessarily went a certain lack of security, though being set in the country five miles away from the nearest village it was isolated from town-based vandals. Nevertheless, there was a continual risk of malicious damage by people bearing ill-will.

A rural setting for a zoo means that many staff people have to live on the premises, and an entity such as Flamingo Park, a little city of keepers, office staff, scientists, showmen, carnival attendants, farmers, maintenance engineers, gardeners, and painters, is a microcosm of society at large, with all the tensions and interplays and aspirations and frustrations of life outside. Where I became involved was when the web of human interactions snared my animal charges. Every day it seemed that one side, either the animals or the humans, got maimed by the other.

The animals usually fared worst. Cases where zoo animals injure humans are usually due to foolhardiness on the part of the human being. Dropping one's guard, becoming cocksure, or taking undue liberties with essentially wild and undomesticated animals usually receives the reward it deserves. There was, for example, the tyro big cat keeper who, after three days in his new occupation, decided to demonstrate his intimacy with the lions and tigers in his care to an admiring group of family friends just up for the day. He reached through the bars and nonchalantly stroked one of his charges; two seconds later, he was minus four fingers.

Another keeper, who ignored repeated warnings against going into the pen with a stallion zebra, fell victim to what I consider to be one of the most dangerous of all animals in the zoo. It happened on a snowy winter's day, and the first notice that I had of it was when the zebra keeper was seen staggering out of the pen having, unbeknown to anyone else, driven off a savage attack by the stallion by ramming snow up its nostrils after it had forced him onto the ground. I happened to be standing in the director's office looking out of the window. "Alf seems to be a bit unsteady on his legs this morning," I said, as I saw the unlucky chap totter slightly as he walked towards the building.

The director came and stood beside me. "He does indeed," he replied, his frown deepening into a pronounced glare. "In fact he's a good deal more than unsteady, he looks drunk. I'll have him in here straight away!"

When the luckless keeper was brought before us, I quickly found him to be in shock rather than inebriated, for although no blood could be seen externally, the power-

ful crushing incisors of a zebra had bitten through his
Wellington boots without rupturing the rubber and produced one of the worst multiple compound fractures of
the ankle that it would be possible to imagine. The bones
had been turned to gravel and exposed and the crucial
Achilles tendon had been severed. The lad never walked
properly again.

Some people never learn, and shortly after coming
back to work fully recovered from the effects of the snake
anti-venom the reptile keeper was faced with yet another
force-feeding task. This time it was a young alligator. I
gave instructions that the animal should have a sort of raw
fondue of dice-sized pieces of steak dipped in a sauce of
beaten raw egg and yeast powder, carefully thrust down
the gullet on the end of a long pair of blunt tweezers. I
emphasized that two people must tackle the job, one to
hold the alligator and one to do the actual feeding. Once
again the reptile keeper elected to do it himself after a
few days of impatience at having to wait for an assistant
from another department to arrive. And once again at
the crucial right-hand left-hand changeover the animal
grabbed him.

This time the wound was high up on the biceps of
his arm. Like all of its kind the alligator bit firmly into the
flesh once and locked its jaws tightly shut. That alone
would not have produced too much damage, unpleasant
as the numerous tooth holes are, particularly as they are
likely to become infected. But, once attached, the reptile
instinctively twisted and lashed its body. In the wild the
leverage produced by this movement wrenches chunks of
meat from the creature held by the traplike jaws. It is this
thrashing that does the real damage. And so it happened
with the reptile keeper's arm. The violent movement of the
alligator's body combined with the firm, well-embedded
grip of its teeth simply pulled the flesh of his upper arm

apart. When I reached him on this occasion, the various bundles of muscles and sinews that surround the humerus bone were peeled apart, separated and displayed as well as on any dissection table, but without the aid of any surgical instruments, let alone a scalpel. The cottage hospital served the fellow well yet again, suturing everything back together under general anaesthetic, but nobody can do anything about the horrible scars which he will bear for the rest of his life.

Sorry as I felt for the human beings in such events, at least they played a crucial part in their own fate. But when things were reversed and humans for one bizarre reason or another wilfully produced suffering for animals, the animals were simply helpless victims.

I was faithful about checking all bolts and padlocks and ensuring that all the animals were secure last thing at night. Despite my vigilance, cranks and vandals occasionally struck successfully. Locks would be sawn through and gates opened to let the animals escape. One can only hazard a guess as to why people do such things. Over the years it has happened two or three dozen times in zoos that I attended, and where the culprits have been apprehended they have turned out to be either teenage delinquents, misguided "anti-zoo" so-called animal lovers, or, once in a while, actual members of the keeping staff. I suppose all of us who work with animals are in some way a little bit nutty, but it is certainly true that there are some strange characters among the zoo-keeping fraternity. Often underpaid and not particularly well treated by senior management, without any sense of involvement in many cases because of the way in which they may be moved willy-nilly from one section of the zoo to another, they can develop deep-seated grudges.

Whoever it was, staff or public, that released stock in

the middle of the night, it was usually my job to go and try to retrieve it. Luckily the species that have been freed have rarely been of the most dangerous sort. I have seen several cases where leopards or lions have got out in zoo gardens, but in almost every case they have caused little or no trouble. Having emerged from the familiar, distinctly bounded territory of their own paddocks and cages, they seem uncertain and apprehensive of the outside world and hole up in a tree or clump of bushes, waiting almost thankfully, I suspect, to be rounded up, darted with the tranquillizer gun, and returned to their quarters.

Sometimes during the high season visitors would actually steal animals to put, I suppose, in their private collections, and I marvel still at the way in which some light-fingered thief went off with a pair of gorgeous eclectus macaws, which had a malevolent distaste for human beings and beaks that could slice like razors, right in the middle of a busy Sunday afternoon. And how did somebody spirit away a porcupine that would wheel and charge backwards, hurling quills at the drop of a hat, or a hawk with talons that could cut through anything but the strongest of leather gloves? They both disappeared on a day when the park was being visited by coachloads of children on school visits. Although the animals were quickly missed and the coaches were searched before they left for home, neither the porcupine nor the hawk was found. However, a three-foot but mercifully docile alligator, whose absence from the pool in the tropical house had gone unobserved, was retrieved from one vehicle, it being found on the back seat wedged firmly under the bottoms of four red-faced little nine-year-olds.

The only animals that actually escaped by their own devices from Flamingo Park were birds. Flamingoes would occasionally fly away for a few days at the seaside, and once a vulture caused consternation among the populace of the little town of Malton by flying in one market day and perching on a telegraph pole in the busy market square to oversee the proceedings.

This problem of zoo birds flying away still faces me from time to time. Traditionally it is tackled by "pinioning," mutilating the bird to permanently remove its gift of flight. A large part of one wing, approximately one third of its length, is cut off. This crippling piece of butchery is frequently done without benefit of any anaesthetic, and not infrequently birds die afterwards from shock or blood loss. When I first went to Flamingo Park I was presented with a newly arrived consignment of storks and cranes and asked to ground them for life. It was a procedure that had never been taught to me at university, although I had watched it performed many times by the head keeper at Belle Vue, and I myself had later pinioned odd birds that had proved themselves to be incorrigible fugitives. The trouble was, I had found the local anaesthetic I injected produced toxic effects in some kinds of bird.

For the storks and cranes at Flamingo Park, I decided to use a new and far less poisonous anaesthetic, but all the same the pile of beautifully feathered pieces on the ground after I had completed my grisly task turned my stomach, and I decided that instead of pinioning zoo birds I would thereafter only feather-clip them. This technique, which is completely painless, simply entails the trimming down with scissors of the primary flight feathers on one wing. When the bird tries to fly, the unbalanced lifting power in the two wings makes it veer to one side and crash on take-off. It soon gets the message and doesn't try any further. It is the best compromise, I suppose, and should last until the birds become accustomed to their new surroundings and lose any desire to escape. But feathers do grow, and in six or nine months the plumage is back to normal again, the bird's power of flight is restored, and some persistent individuals will be on their way unless one remembers to clip their feathers again.

Man's inhumanity to animals has many aspects. For me one of the most tragic incidents involved some highly trained performing parrots which pulled large crowds during the summer season at Flamingo Park. The clever, brilliantly coloured birds had an amazing repertoire of tricks, ranging from riding a unicycle across a tightrope to firing candy bars from a cannon, from roller skating and cycling to driving an electric motorcar. They played cards with members of the audience and demonstrated a remarkable talent for Find the Lady. Trained by kindness to work for rewards of peanuts, and with robust trouble-free constitutions, they were easy to keep and rarely appeared on my daily sick parade. They really were a professional little band of troupers, keeping themselves to themselves in their cages in a special wooden hut behind the scenes when not on duty, and sitting like showgirls on their perches in the sunshine when waiting for their turn in the limelight.

One night I was sleeping in my trailer about a mile from the animal houses when something wakened me. It was a strange dull thud. I felt instinctively alarmed and, opening the curtains, peered out of the little window. In the distance there was a reddish glow in the moonless black of the sky, a glow centred right over the middle of the complex of zoo buildings. Something was on fire! Pulling on some trousers I dashed outside to my car and drove with a pounding heart towards the area of sinister light.

When I arrived I found the wooden parrot house to be

already a blazing inferno. The thud which had wakened me had been the explosion of a gas cylinder kept on the premises as a source of winter fuel. When the flames reached it, it had gone up, intensifying the blaze and shattering the interior of the building.

A crowd of staff had gathered and was vainly trying to control the conflagration. The girl who trained the birds was weeping hysterically and had to be forcibly restrained from rushing into the shed to try to save some of the poor parrots. The fire brigade arrived and began running out their hoses. It seemed like hours before the flames at last died down and it was possible to enter what was left of the building. I have never seen a more pitiful sight. In each twisted and blackened cage lay the remains of a bird. Twelve parrots had perished by suffocation or from burning, some of them no more than charred husks. Miraculously, one of the parrots had survived the holocaust. With barely a feather left on his blackened and blistered little body, he lay gasping on his side on the smoking floor of the cage. A scooter rider of dash and polish who had always been antipathetic towards me, he had led his companions in a deafening chorus of raucous jeers whenever I had looked them over at the weekly health inspection. Now he was the most agonized creature I have ever seen.

I carefully lifted him out and took him into the cool night air. Holding him seemed to burn the palms of my hands, and I could feel the feeble little heart beat faster than seemed possible. His beak gaped wide as he gasped desperately to drag air into lungs and air sacs that had been seared by the fiery vapours. Listening with my stethoscope I could hear the fluid that would drown him beginning to rise in his chest. I began to calculate what, if anything, I could do for him. Oxygen? Steroids? Take him to my surgery? At that moment the baked and bleeding little eyelids opened a fraction, and I caught a glimpse of the familiar cheeky bright eye observing me. As I looked down at the parrot the eye fixed me and then followed me as I turned my head to speak to someone standing nearby. The eye that had been so mischievous and wicked during the good days now seemed somehow benign and imploring.

There was only one thing that I could do for him. Handing him over carefully to the zoo director, I fetched a bottle of barbiturate injection from my car. A minute later the suffering bird dropped into a bottomless sleep.

While the fire was being put out we discovered that other parts of the zoo were also alight. An arsonist had been at work. Police investigations revealed that the culprit was an elephant keeper. At his trial it turned out that he had had a disagreement with the assistant director and as a result had wreaked his vengeance not on the elephants but on the parrots and, without success, on the zebras and Ankole cattle.

7 A Wild Goose in Pakistan

DURING MY TENURE as curator at Flamingo Park, the expansion of Pentland Hick's little empire of zoos and leisure parks was at its peak. The company was particularly interested in marine mammals, and every week new specimens would be brought in or expeditions to find others would be planned or set into operation. I became a one-man expedition myself shortly after I had completed my year and a half's stint at the park and had returned to Rochdale to take care of my growing practice.

"Can you go out straight away to Pakistan?" Pentland Hick asked, terse as usual, one morning as we stood together watching the king penguins taking their first dip of the day. "There's a chap near the border with Afghanistan who claims he's got pygmy sperm whales."

Kogia breviceps, the pygmy sperm whale, is a charming miniaturization of the cachalot or sperm whale. Never growing much above seven feet in length, as compared to the sperm whale's length of fifty to sixty feet, it appears to be widely distributed throughout the oceans of the world, although it is very rarely seen by man. It tends to swim alone or in small groups and feeds on squid and probably crabs. Virtually nothing is known about its habits or reproduction, but because it is small, weighing only 600 to 700 pounds, and therefore easy to transport, and because it has teeth and prefers food which is readily available in Britain, it was a suitable and exciting prospect for Hick's expanding collection of killer whales and other cetaceans. Two other small whales on which we were working at the time, the beluga and the narwhal, need refrigeration equipment to keep the temperature of their pool down to arctic levels. *Kogia* seemed to be a frequenter of much more temperate waters and therefore easier to keep.

The man who had written to Hick with the offer of pygmy sperm whales was unknown to us. He was apparently a Scottish naturalist living in Quetta, the provincial capital of Baluchistan, and dealt in birds and animals of that part of the world which he claimed to supply to zoos in various countries. His name, let us say, was McPherson. Apart from friends at the Steinhart Aquarium in San Francisco, who said that they had met a man of that name while collecting fresh-water dolphins in Pakistan some weeks earlier, I could find no one in the zoo or animal business who had heard of him. Still, his letter stated plainly and without ambiguity that he had *Kogia breviceps* for sale and at a reasonable price.

"I want you to go out as soon as possible and see what McPherson has got to offer," said Hick. "We can't afford to run the risk of anyone else in Europe beating us to it."

As soon as possible was the next day. I booked my flight to Karachi by radio telephone while driving back from Flamingo Park to Rochdale. One thing that puzzled me when I got home and consulted the atlas was that Quetta is situated hundreds of miles from the sea in the rugged hills of the north-west frontier—an unusual base for whale-catching. I could not recall any reference to such goings-on in those stirring films that featured Errol Flynn and his lancers.

I flew out to Karachi via Moscow on Pakistan International Airways, a thoroughly miserable flight; within thirty minutes of leaving Heathrow almost all the passengers had been air-sick. After a brief rest in Karachi I took off again for Quetta, this time in a small, rather ancient aeroplane. The passenger sitting next to me was a pleasant but loquacious character with a brother in England whom, he felt sure, I must have met. He was carrying a block of what looked like fudge wrapped in silver paper and weighing about three pounds. It was high-quality cannabis resin, mine to take home as a souvenir for a mere £20, my companion suggested. After all, he posted it regularly to his brother in Birmingham. I tried to disengage from the conversation by concentrating on the view through the aircraft window as we flew north over red desert country, but my neighbour had not finished with me yet. After downing the best part of a pint of whisky from a bottle he produced from his bag, he was apologetically sick all over my trousers. The Pakistan adventure was not beginning well.

The red desert suddenly gave way to a mountainous grey lunar landscape. Valleys and peaks looked uniformly sterile and forbidding, unrelieved by any streams or trees or signs of habitation. As we came in to land at the airfield which serves Quetta, the resemblance to the moon's surface was even more striking. We glided down onto a grim grey plateau, the centre of a vast crater in the middle of the mountains. Apart from a small building that served as the air terminal, nothing but pallid dust could be seen in any direction.

Having collected my bags and discovered that the hotel in Quetta to which PIA in Manchester had cabled to reserve a room for me had been pulled down five years earlier, I found myself standing alone in the dust outside the terminal wondering where to go and how. Apparently there was no way of getting into the town, some miles away. Apart from the man in the tiny control tower, who did not seem interested in opening his door or window to discover what it was I kept shouting at him, there was no one about. The aircraft had taken off for its next destination, Peshawar, and light was beginning to fade.

Just then a decrepit old station wagon came rattling down the road. It was tightly packed with fierce-looking Pathans and an assortment of skinny goats and sheep. Desperate to get moving, I ran out into the road and flagged the vehicle down. It stopped and I scrambled thankfully into the tight press of smelly animals. The men said not a word to me and hardly cast a glance in my direction. It was as if they had not noticed the addition to their load. We rumbled off in clouds of dust and eventually arrived at the town. When the wagon stopped in a narrow street of dilapidated wooden shacks and stinking open sewers, I got out and thanked the driver, who drove on without acknowledging my farewells in any way. By this time I was very dishevelled and reeked of an outlandish mixture of human vomit and goat.

It was a long time before I found someone who spoke English and who could direct me to the only hotel in Quetta, a decaying wooden relic of the British Empire called, of all things, the Regina Coeli. An unprepossessing character, unshaven and with a wall-eye, who spoke a little English, informed me that I would be their sole guest and showed me to the filthiest suite of rooms I have ever seen.

Darkness had fallen and it had grown bitterly cold. My host brought a home-made metal stove and set it up in my room. He explained its intricacies and temperamental ways and sold me a quantity of oil for it at an astronomical price. By the light of its noisy, fluctuating flame I was able, once I was alone, to explore the four rooms I had been given, including a lavatory built directly over an evil cesspit. There were doors everywhere, behind which I could hear people shuffling about and murmuring. Whoever they were, they seemed to be constantly on the thresholds at the other side of the doors. It was eerie and disturbing. With much difficulty, for apart from a low wooden bed and the stove there was not a scrap of furniture in the rooms, I secured all the doors by wedging bits of wood or stone under them, closed the shutters and wired them so that they could not be opened from outside, and went to bed.

As I lay on the low bed I noticed an irregular pattern of red dots decorating the crumbling white plaster of the walls. It was difficult to tell what they were by the light of the stove, so I struck a match for closer inspection. They were the bloody patches where countless fingers had squashed bedbugs into oblivion. I could see thumbprints and the fragments of corpses ground into the plaster. Dismayed, I got up and took the cowl off the stove. The flames soared up to the ceiling and coated it with oily soot. Now I could see better. I had never actually met *Cimex lectularius*, the bedbug, in person, but I had studied him and his kind when doing my Fellowship and knew where he was likely to be found. Sure enough, from the dry rot of the skirting board and from wide cracks in the wall plaster, like climbers from a rock chimney, the flat and unmistakable insects were beginning to emerge. I stripped the bed and found and eradicated more of them. Finally, with oil from the stove I made shallow pools on the stone floor round the bed legs and painted a strip of oil round all four walls to prevent my unwelcome companions from climbing up to the ceiling and launching parachute attacks. Exhausted and miserable, cold and damp, still smelling of goat and other things, I eventually fell asleep fully clothed on top of the bed.

A peep into the kitchen the following morning made

me decide to fast for as long as I was in the hotel, and
hunger was now added to my miseries. The cook thought
it most strange that I would take nothing but tea, and that
without milk, but I was reluctant to share a repast with the
two enormous brown rats that I had just seen sitting in a
cooling pan of vegetables, eating unhurriedly from the
warm pottage in which they reclined.

My job was to find McPherson and his pygmy sperm
whales and then to get out of Quetta with all speed, but this
proved to be almost impossible. The hotel owner knew of
no Englishman or Scot with such a name in the town. He
could not think of any Europeans in the place at all, except
for the strange young people who passed through from
time to time on their way from Afghanistan to India:
Quetta is a watering-place on the twentieth-century pil-
grims' way.

I went into town past the derelict barracks and rusting cannon still bearing the names of famous British regi-
ments, down streets lined by windowless wooden dwellings
as small as police boxes and with sacks for doors, and across
weedy fields where white mosques gleamed against the
grey backdrop of the mountains. Quetta looks like a
frontier town, which, in fact, it is. It was devastated by an
earthquake in 1935 and has never recovered. I found the
police station, the office of the agriculture ministry, and
the municipal headquarters. No one had heard of McPherson or, indeed, of any naturalists working in the area. As
for whales, even the English-speaking people that I met
did not understand the meaning of the word. When I
drew a picture of a whale to make matters clearer their
eyes opened wide and they looked at me curiously. "But
the sea is far away, sir," said one puzzled policeman.

All day I wandered through the town looking for
clues to the whereabouts of McPherson. Knots of tall,

striking-looking Baluch tribesmen standing on the corners found me an object of great curiosity and some amusement as I tried to orient myself with the aid of a street map of 1940 vintage. McPherson's letter naturally bore an address. Not only could I not find the street on my map, but no one I spoke to admitted any knowledge of such a place. The day ended with me no nearer finding the elusive naturalist, but my hunger was growing and the weather was becoming colder, threatening rain. I spent another unhappy night at the hotel fortified only by tea and lay awake most of the night as a great storm swept down from the mountains and the wind threatened to blow the building away.

Off I went round the town again the next morning. I was becoming convinced that McPherson was some sort of confidence trickster trying to extract money by false pretences from Pentland Hick. Perhaps he had been hoping to obtain a deposit in advance. But in that case why pick on Quetta as a supposed base for his marine operations? And if the address was false, as seemed likely, how could money sent by mail possibly reach him? I decided to try the post office again. The day before I had drawn a blank, but surely if the man or his address had ever existed in Quetta he must have received mail.

I had gone into the post office building and stood looking at the rows of numbered boxes when someone tapped me on my shoulder. I looked round to find a large, smartly dressed policeman with a swagger stick confronting me.

"Dr. Taylor, sir?" he inquired politely. "I wonder if you would be kind enough to come with me. My superintendent would like to meet you."

He led me out to his jeep. A fat man with bloodshot eyes and a nude blonde painted on his tie sat silently in the back seat. We bounced through the rough, rubble-strewn streets and stopped outside a tall building covered with peeling pink paint. The policeman led me inside and the fat man followed behind. We entered an office where another policeman sat at a desk and a civilian wearing gumboots sat on a settee against one wall. The man behind the desk smiled, introduced himself as the superintendent, and asked me to sit down. This must be something to do with the guy on the plane, I thought, my sick friend with the cannabis.

"Dr. Taylor, I have asked you to come in to see us," the superintendent began, "because we believe you are having difficulties finding an acquaintance of yours."

Very civil, I thought. Perhaps they have located him for me. "Yes," I said, "Mr. McPherson, the naturalist."

The man with bloodshot eyes grunted loudly. There was silence for a few moments.

"McPherson, the naturalist." The superintendent repeated my words slowly, as if reflecting on them. "Are you here to see him on business or on pleasure?"

"Business. I'm up here to see him about whales. I'm a veterinary surgeon."

Now the fat bloodshot individual grunted again and spoke for the first time. "Dr. Taylor, a veterinary surgeon, eh? An animal doctor from England, eh? To see McPherson the naturalist, eh?"

"Yes indeed," I replied, beginning to feel a little uneasy. "Why? Is there something odd about that?"

The superintendent spoke again. "This is Major Darwish," he said, indicating the fat man. "Major Darwish of Military Security."

For the next hour I sat while Major Darwish explained the reason for this interview. There was political trouble in Baluchistan, moves for regional autonomy, even secession. It was a sensitive area, with border problems, big-power interest, and so on. The Pakistan government had detected American CIA activity in the border area, based on Quetta. Some Americans had been asked to leave the country, and McPherson was thought to be implicated in the whole business.

"We've got our eye on your Mr. McPherson," said Major Darwish, "and we've got our eye on anyone who comes up here trying to fish in troubled waters. The tribal problems are delicate enough for Karachi without foreigners making matters worse." He leaned forward towards me and spoke in a mock confidential tone. "Do you know Quetta has been crawling with CIA men?"

The penny dropped. I had been hauled in as a possible agent of a foreign power!

"You don't think I'm a CIA man, do you?" I laughed, perhaps a shade too heartily.

There was silence; then the superintendent said, "But we are told, Dr. Taylor, that you are an animal doctor looking for a man who has whales, that you have been inquiring around town as to where he lives and saying to people that you are here to inspect sea animals. We do not have whales or sea animals in Quetta. The sea is far away. And we are wishing to assure ourselves that what you tell us is right."

"It is right," I said with some annoyance. "That's why I'm here."

"We would like to be sure that you are indeed an animal doctor," cut in Darwish. "What university did you attend?"

I gave them a terse curriculum vitae and finished by saying that if they would produce a horse or a goat for a demonstration of my trade I would prove I was telling the truth by castrating it neatly on the spot.

"Well," said Darwish, "that won't be necessary. This gentleman is Dr. Mohammed, a veterinary graduate of Lahore who works in the government service here." He pointed to the man sitting silently on the settee in his gum-

boots. "I think Dr. Mohammed might ask you a couple of
questions to validate your claim to be a veterinary surgeon.
I'm sure you will understand."

I was stunned. Here was I, suspected of being a spy in
the fastnesses of the north-west frontier, about to be given
a viva voce by another vet about whom I knew nothing.
What if he had firm but erroneous opinions on some matter
on which he questioned me? And was there not a good
chance that he would ask me about some local malady about
which I knew little or nothing?

Dr. Mohammed stood up importantly and cleared his
throat. "Now, sir," he began, with an air of great solemnity,
"would you kindly answer the following three questions.
Firstly, what is the volume of the gall-bladder in the mule?
Secondly, for what do I use butter of antimony? And
thirdly, what is Bang's disease?"

He sat down with a satisfied smile. Everyone looked
at me. The first question was a trick one.

"Well, Dr. Mohammed," I said, "the answer to the one
about the gall-bladder of the mule is that its volume is
exactly the same as that of the dolphin's gall-bladder."

Dr. Mohammed jumped to his feet with gleaming eyes.
"Aha," he exclaimed, somewhat theatrically, "you really
will have to be more explicit than that. I asked you the
volume. Approximately how many cc's?"

"Like I said, the same as a dolphin's or, in other words,
zero." Horses and mules and whales and dolphins do not
possess gall-bladders, although they do produce bile and
have bile ducts.

Mohammed sat down again, looking a trifle crestfallen.

"The second question about butter of antimony is a
bit old-fashioned," I continued. "I've not seen it used for
years, but it was applied to foot infections in cattle. Bang's
disease is contagious brucella abortion."

There was another long silence and then Darwish began a lengthy questioning of Dr. Mohammed in Urdu. Eventually he turned to me.

"Dr. Taylor, you may go; we are satisfied. We wish you well in your search for Mr. McPherson."

"But I assume you know where he is," I said. "You say you're keeping an eye on him. How do I find him?"

"I'm sorry," replied the superintendent. "He was here, but we don't know where he is now."

Everyone looked a bit sheepish and I realized that my interview was over and that I was not going to get any more out of them. Thanking them, I left the building and took a bicycle rickshaw back to the hotel. I would leave next morning for Karachi. McPherson had been the cause of a wild goose chase. Pygmy sperm whales indeed!

The hotel keeper said that there would be no flights out on the following day. The storms were still blowing in the mountains and small aircraft could not make it over the high peaks encircling the town. In low spirits I sat in my room drinking tea, hungrier than ever. Somehow I felt that it might be worth one more try at finding McPherson, especially as I would have to spend at least another day in this dreary place anyway.

The next morning dawned grey and showery. Walking down into the town I puzzled over where to make more inquiries. As I stood looking round, a sign on a small bungalow across the road caught my eye. "Ministry of Forests," it read. Perhaps they knew of naturalists going on expeditions in areas under their supervision. I went in and asked the first person I saw for the director. He got my meaning and took me through dim corridors cluttered with ragged figures squatting in corners and against walls. The Director of Forestry was a pleasant little man who spoke some English. To my delight, when I brought up the

question of McPherson the naturalist, I did not receive the
expected blank look and shake of the head.

"I think I know who you mean," he said. "I'm not certain of the name but there is an Englishman." He rang a bell
and an assistant appeared. "I'll get Hussein here to take
you."

I was elated. It looked as if I had done it at last.
Hussein hailed a bicycle rickshaw and we climbed in.
Through the middle of the town we went, and into an area
which I had not explored on foot. The streets became nar-
rower and the tarmac gave way to dirt tracks between
tightly packed wooden hovels. We rattled through a maze
of muddy lanes where beggars crouched over open sewers
and thin dogs covered with sores barked and howled. We
were in the worst of the slums, surely the wrong place.

Abruptly we came upon the only proper building in
the middle of that odorous shanty town, a dirty white
bungalow that had known far better days and was surrounded by a high wall of dried mud. We stopped and paid
off the rickshaw driver and knocked on the gate. After
much barking of dogs it opened and a young man in baggy
trousers whom I took to be a house-boy let us in. I explained why we were there and he took us into the house.

Inside it was dim and smoky. We were led into a large
room that looked like a curio shop. Stuffed animals were
piled round the walls, trinkets and weapons and articles of
falconry equipment hung in clusters from the ceiling.
Three hawks sat on blocks in the middle of the stone floor.
In the light of the log fire, lying on a sofa drawn up close
to the hearth, lay a European of about forty with tangled
hair and a reddish beard. He was sleeping fully dressed in
grubby clothes. His face was covered in big drops of sweat
and his hands and arms were a mass of nasty sores. The
house-boy gently roused the sleeping figure, who opened
his eyes but made no attempt to rise.

"Good morning," I said, as he blinked at me and wiped his eyes feebly. "I'm Dr. Taylor from Flamingo Park, England. Are you McPherson, by any chance?"

In a polished public-school accent he replied, "I am, but I'm afraid I'm not well at present. You shouldn't have come out here until I asked you to come."

His voice was weak and tired. The sores on his arms were going septic and the lymphatic channels stood out in dull red lines. I asked him what was wrong. Apparently he had been severely bitten by some falcons and was obviously at least on the brink of septicaemia. I always carry a selection of broad-spectrum antibiotics when visiting the East, so I gave him all the terramycin tablets I had. He accepted them gratefully. Apparently antibiotics were hard to come by and expensive, and it was clear that he was very short of cash. I told him I would give the antibiotics time to take effect and start reducing his fever, then I would return later in the day and talk with him.

After spending the day in the foothills outside the town I returned alone to McPherson's house with the aid of a scrap of paper on which his house-boy had written the directions for the rickshaw driver. McPherson was looking a bit better, sitting up and dressing his wounds. I got straight down to brass tacks—I had come to see his pygmy sperm whales.

He had problems there, it appeared. The whales were six hundred miles away by the coast. Could I go down to see them? No, because he hadn't known I was arriving and would be unable to accompany me. Alone, then? Well, no, that would be difficult.

I began to realize that my whole trip had been in vain. As we talked I found him anxious to discuss the financial aspects of the matter and keen to describe how he had trapped the animals, but as I pressed him to tell me precisely how many whales he actually had and exactly where, it became clear that he had none. Nor did his catching facilities and holding pools seem to have much substance. He showed me photographs of seascapes and muddy estuaries, but on none were there any traces of sea mammals. The pictures could have been taken anywhere.

He was adamant that he could not accompany me to the coast.

"I shall go alone, then, and look around for myself," I said.

"If only you had waited until I told you to come," McPherson replied, "I could have shown you pygmy sperms."

He could not explain why his letter had so enthusiastically assured customers that the whales were ready and waiting for inspection. I asked him about Major Darwish and the CIA. He agreed that some of his friends had been expelled and showed me the Land Rover they had had to leave behind, but he was reluctant to talk further about the matter or to tell me how and why he existed in such an odd place. Apart from the dogs and hawks, there were no animals to be seen or heard.

Before I left to pack my bags, McPherson said there was something else I might be interested in. What would Pentland Hick offer for a pair of giant pandas? It is impossible to put a price on this most popular and rare of exotic animals, but I said that I was sure he would give a million pounds. McPherson had a scheme, on which he was shortly to embark, for smuggling pandas out of China. Would I like to join the expedition?

The plan was breathtaking. A team of men, including me as vet to tranquillize the animals and watch their health, would leave East Pakistan and travel by mule and on foot across Assam, skirt the foothills of the Nyenchentanglha Mountains of Tibet, and reach the panda country of

Szechwan in China. The distance was about 850 miles over high, uninhabited regions for the second half of the journey. The pandas would be brought back into Pakistan, dyed brown, and shipped out as low-value brown bears. McPherson showed me the maps and other documents he had collected in preparation for the expedition.

"Will you join us?" he asked. "It would be worth twenty-five thousand pounds to you."

"I'll wait until we've got some pygmy sperm whales first," I said. "Then I might consider it."

Two days later the weather improved and I took a flight back to Karachi. My normally robust constitution had wilted noticeably on a diet of nothing but tea. After four days of fasting the pangs of hunger had been numbed, but they returned in a trice as I dashed into the bar of the Intercontinental Hotel and downed surely the most ambrosial gin and tonic man had up to that time concocted. Then, without stopping to check into my room, take a shower, or otherwise ameliorate my malodorous and dishevelled condition, I hurried up to the swanky roof-top restaurant. There, in glittering gowns and sharkskin tuxedos, the upper crust of Pakistani society was elegantly circulating around a long and heavily loaded buffet set in the middle of the room.

With the urgency of an eagle of the kind I had seen swooping over Quetta, I moved in and filled a tray with mounds of spiced lamb, curried duck, tandoori-cooked fish, stuffed aubergines, lobster roasted with apricots, and a wobbling stack of *nan*, the hot fresh-baked local muffins. Oblivious to the disdainful regard of the head waiter, I gorged myself at a table situated close to the buffet so as to be within easy reach of second, third, and fourth helpings. I was restored.

The next day I decided to visit the fishing villages on

the coastline near the city to see what the fishermen knew
about sea mammals in the area. I visited a number of primi-
tive fishing communities on the salt flats north-west and
south of the city, accompanied by a helpful employee of
the Dutch airline KLM, whose reputation for transporting animals is superb. I took with me a book of coloured
illustrations of various species of sea mammals. The fact that
the labelling and text was all in Japanese did not matter, as
the man from KLM asked the fishermen just to point to
pictures of any animals that they had encountered. Men at
every village nodded when I pointed to the spinner dolphin. Some knew the pilot whale and the killer. At only
one village could I find a man who had apparently seen a
pygmy sperm whale, and that only in deep water and very
infrequently.

They smiled and nodded at pictures of the dugong,
probable origin of the mermaid myth. Yes, they were well
acquainted with her, and was she not a cross between man
and dolphin? In one village the dugong picture brought
much shuffling of feet and embarrassed lowering of heads.
The KLM man said that they knew of fishermen who had
taken dugongs as lovers, but that they did not like to
talk about it with strangers. Dugongs were trouble. Their
wives would scold them for days if they knew that they
had even discussed them.

So pygmy sperm whales were not to be. Before leaving
Karachi for home I cabled McPherson to say that there was
nothing doing at the coast. Just before I left my hotel to go
to the airport he telephoned me from Quetta saying that
he had some more of the elusive creatures in a set of ponds
about twenty miles east of Karachi. If only I would wait a
few days I would see.

I told him I had to depart, and bade him farewell.

I have not heard any more from McPherson, nor to my

knowledge has anyone else. About pygmy sperm whales in Pakistan we are no wiser, although some three months after I returned there arrived at Flamingo Park an unsigned cable that read PLEASE SEND FORTY YARDS STRONG TAPE FOR CONSTRUCTING CARRYING SLINGS PYGMY SPERMS URGENT. The telegraph office of origin was Quetta.

8 The Feast of Saint Sylvestre

URGENT CALLS FROM ABROAD have a knack of coming in on the eve of highdays and holidays, as if part of some grand design to keep me from ever taking a break. Almost every year Christmas, Easter, and New Year's Day find me in some outlandish spot being cordially welcomed into the local festivities after I have examined and treated the animals that are the object of my visit, when my working clothes of old shirt and jeans are black with dust from a rhinoceros or sodden with sea water.

Some weeks after my return from Pakistan I was asked to go immediately to a city in France on New Year's Eve, the feast of Saint Sylvestre, to give my opinion of a seriously ill bottle-nosed dolphin. One of the great things about living in Rochdale is that it lies roughly at the centre of the British Isles and is well served by motorways and a first-class international airport in Manchester twenty minutes away, with direct connections to capitals on the continent. I was on the plane to France within three hours of the telephone call. As usual, to avoid delay at the baggage claim or customs, I carried all my drugs and instruments and enough clothes for a two- or three-day stay as hand baggage in a holdall. On the plane I as usual selected an aisle seat on the front row nearest to the door, so that

I could deplane fast and be first of the bunch through immigration and away. If people think it's worth-while sending for me from hundreds or thousands of miles away, I owe it to them to be fleet of foot. I reckon that my chances of success, and possibly the life of an animal, can swing on every minute that can be saved.

It was my first visit to this particular zoo, and I arrived in the evening just after dark. Godot, the director and owner of the zoo, was waiting to pick me up. From the look of the gleaming Citroën S.M. that he had with him I felt sure it would not take long to cover the seventeen miles from airport to zoo. But it wasn't going to be quite so easy. Godot shook my hand, murmured some words of welcome, and then gestured towards a small group of men standing to one side, clutching large cameras.

"Perhaps before we set off, Dr. Taylor," he said, "you would not mind just letting these photographers take a picture and make a few notes. The local papers, you know. They have been very interested in the troubles of our sick dolphin, Nicki. Good public relations, I think."

The press men descended upon us. Flash bulbs popped, and they all asked me questions at one and the same time in French.

"Can't all this wait until I've had a chance to examine the dolphin?" I asked, somewhat testily. "Why don't they wait until I know what I'm talking about?"

But there was no putting them off. M. Godot shrugged his shoulders but said that it would only take a few minutes. He didn't speak much English, and my French wilted under the onslaught of half a dozen simultaneously gabbled questions in the local patois. All over the world dolphins and their ailments are accorded publicity treatment more usually given to pop stars or film actresses. They are truly showbiz animals.

Eventually we got away but we had lost twenty min-

utes. As we travelled in towards the city M. Godot outlined Nicki's troubles. The dolphin had been ill for about
two weeks and had lost much weight. In the past forty-
eight hours he had gone completely off his food. No one
had been able to pinpoint exactly what was wrong, and he
had been treated by homoeopathy.

I had never previously actually come in contact with
cases of animals being treated under this system of medicine. I had read about the theory of "like treats like," the
administration of minute doses of chemicals whose effects
are similar to those produced by the symptoms of the
disease under treatment. (A good example would be the
prescribing of very tiny amounts of strychnine, a poison
that produces convulsive spasms, in the treatment of
tetanus, a disease characterized by convulsive spasms.)
Years ago homoeopathy in animal medicine had a small
body of adherents in Great Britain, but I hadn't heard of it
for years. It apparently still lingered on in French veterinary medicine, however, and in this case had consisted of
giving the animal amounts of garlic crushed with rock salt.
Despite this savoury treatment, the dolphin's condition had
gravely worsened. But no one had caught the animal and
examined him closely with hands and ears and eyes, nor
had any blood been taken for laboratory analysis.

Eventually we turned in to the small zoological gardens set in the heart of the city. It was an old-fashioned
place with many cages whose ancient iron bars were wider
than the free spaces between them, making it difficult to
catch more than a glimpse of the inmates beyond. It had
begun to pour down with rain, and M. Godot hurried me
into one of the buildings. It was the restaurant.

"Come, Dr. Taylor," he said. "I'm sure you're ready
for dinner after your long journey."

He introduced me to a small group of his assistants

who were waiting for us in the otherwise deserted dining room. As it was out of season the place had obviously been specially opened for the New Year's celebration, and a chef hovered expectantly on the threshold of the kitchen door. A long table set with a number of bottles of wine and small dishes of olives and raw vegetables had been laid in the middle of the room.

I have always made it a rule no matter what the hour or how long the journey to make at least a preliminary examination of the patient before eating, drinking, or relaxing in any other way. "I think I would prefer to go and see the dolphin now, rather than later," I said. "The sooner we can get cracking the better. Could we not eat later?"

The Frenchmen raised their eyebrows, pursed their lips, and looked at one another. "I think it would be better if we ate now. It's raining heavily and the dolphin pool is an outdoor one. There's no moon tonight and you wouldn't be able to see a thing. Yes, I'm sure it would be better to eat now." M. Godot shook his head slowly and spread his hands palms upward in an apologetic gesture.

"Nevertheless, I've come a long way today to see this dolphin, and he sounds as if he's very ill." I was feeling a bit grumpy by this time. "I can have a look at him perfectly well with artificial light."

"But there is no light at the pool side, I'm afraid, Dr. Taylor."

"No light?" What nonsense, I thought. "Can't you run a cable from the nearest electric point and fit me up with a bulb or something?"

Everyone began talking rapidly in French. I could just about gather the gist of what it was all about. Two things were clear. One, I was running the risk of making myself unpopular, and two, no one felt like setting up the cable and lamp in the darkness and the rain. The more they debated, the more adamant I became. I was determined to insist that they should do me the courtesy, now that I had gone to a great deal of trouble to arrive without delay, to provide me with ample help in taking the first look over my patient. Eventually it was decided that someone would go to look for a cable and suitable bulb.

"Mathieu has gone to see what he can do," said M. Godot. "He will be back shortly. Please, while we wait at least have an aperitif."

Well, I thought, it shouldn't take more than five minutes. There was no harm in having a Pernod while I waited, so we all sat down while a waiter prepared a round of drinks.

Mathieu returned in twenty-five minutes. He was looking disconsolate and very damp. He announced with much gesticulation that the dolphin pool would have to remain lightless. Of that he was certain. A cable he had, but a bulb to fit the socket on the end of the cable he had not. There wasn't such a bulb to be found in the whole of the zoo! *Oui, s'il vous plait,* he would have a jigger of Pastis on the rocks!

"But there must be some way of getting a simple light bulb to the edge of the pool so that I can have a look at the dolphin," I protested. "This is a serious matter. I must have the pool illuminated."

Everyone began to talk excitedly at the same time but with voices pitched an octave higher than before. Another supportive round of aperitifs was dispensed.

"I have come to treat an emergency on Saint Sylvestre's! Why can I not examine my patient?" I kept on repeating in what I hoped was intelligible French. *"Pourquoi? Pourquoi?"*

It was decided that Mathieu would be sent into the town to find a suitable bulb. Of course the shops would be

closed, but if I could be patient no doubt he would be able
to find one somewhere, and all would be well. Mathieu
left and it was suggested to me it really would be a good
idea to have dinner in the interim. Reluctantly I agreed and
the repast began.

What a meal it turned out to be! First came trays full
of succulent small French oysters accompanied by chilled
white wines from the Loire. Then there was bouillabaisse,
the exquisite fish soup of southern France, on which
floated croutons basted with garlic and fiery mustard, followed by vast bowls of a luscious *salade niçoise*. A whole
poached salmon, beautifully glazed and decorated with
capers, lemon, and mayonnaise came next, then tender
steaks of veal with chanterelles, crêpes in Grand Marnier,
a magnificent cheese board, and fresh fruits. The whole
meal was consumed at a most leisurely pace. I was introduced to some outstanding varieties of Provençal wines.

Of Mathieu there was no sign. "No matter," said my
companions. "It is a very unpleasant night outside. It is
sure to be a much better day in the morning." What was
more, they had a special treat in store for me! When the
fruit had been consumed, M. Godot clicked his fingers and
the chef proudly advanced towards the table bearing an
enormous gâteau on a tray. It had been made in the shape
of a dolphin and was really quite a masterpiece, with ic-
ing of an accurate if not very appetizing grey colour.
Everyone was most pleased with this culinary high spot,
and lashings of iced champagne were poured to wash it
down.

Just as I was cutting the cake to the polite applause of
the other diners and debating within myself whether I
should be annoyed or amused by this ridiculous situation
which had substituted gastronomy for medicine, friend
Mathieu returned. There was a grim air of finality about

him. It was finished. No bulbs of the correct fitting could
he find. That was that. The Frenchmen agreed. In no way,
regrettably, was it going to be possible for me to do much
until day broke, so on with the excellent coffee and balloon
glasses of Armagnac. I was very disappointed, but one
glance through the window showed me that visibility in the
deep black night was zero.

I was sitting quietly ruminating over my coffee when
a newcomer arrived. It was one of the reporters who had
interviewed me at the airport. He hoped he wasn't too late
to take some action pictures of me examining Nicki.
Naturally he was carrying his camera with him and I
noticed an electronic flash gun. Well, I wondered, looking
at his equipment, would it be possible? It might just work in
a fashion.

So it came about that a few minutes later I was standing in my raincoat on the edge of the dolphin pool while the
rain teemed down and the reporter aimed his flash gun at the
water, firing it repeatedly. For an instant lasting perhaps a
hundredth of a second I had a glimpse of the creature that
I had come so far to see lying listlessly in the water, his eyes
glowing red in the magnesium flare. *Click!* And for a trice
I had an impression of an emaciated dolphin with ugly
angles and bumps where his skeleton was jutting through
the depleted layers of blubber. *Click!* I tried to imprint the
image of the animal on my visual memory so that I
could take a considered look at the condition of the skin
and the colour of the mucous membranes. *Click!* Always the light failed to coincide with the taking of a breath
and the opening of the blow hole. *Click!* The dolphin had
gone spiraling down somewhere beneath the dark water.

What a way to examine an animal. At least I had seen
Nicki, but it was impossible to give even a preliminary
opinion about him, and catching him was certainly out of

the question. I went back to the restaurant and asked what time we could begin the following day.

"What time would you like to start, Dr. Taylor?"

"How about six thirty A.M.?"

There was silence and some shuffling of feet.

"Seven o'clock?" I suggested, improving my offer. Everyone still looked glum. "What about eight o'clock then?" Still I had no takers. "Eight thirty, can anyone help me to take him out at eight thirty?" I asked in desperation.

At last they brightened up a little and someone replied, "Certainly, Dr. Taylor, you will have all the help you need tomorrow. . . . How about nine o'clock?"

So the poor dolphin had only another eleven hours to go before I could begin trying to do something for him. I went off to a hotel for the night and welcomed the New Year alone in my room and in low spirits. I didn't see what else I could have done, but whether I liked it or not I felt I had let the animal down. We all had. I fell asleep thinking how such a fiasco could never have happened in a country such as Germany, where I've always found everything organized down to the finest detail whenever I have arrived.

The next morning, M. Godot telephoned my hotel to say that he was sending a vehicle and chauffeur to pick me up. After breakfast I went out of the foyer of the hotel onto the busy main thoroughfare. There was M. Godot in his car, but parked directly in front of the hotel steps was a motorcycle, and waiting patiently on the driving seat, dressed in sweater, trousers, and peaked cap, was a large and unconcerned-looking chimpanzee.

"Get on the pillion seat behind Henri," M. Godot shouted from the car when I appeared. "He is a good driver!"

The zoo was a mile or more away, and we would have to go through the traffic-choked centre of the city to get there. I consider myself a reasonably competent driver in most European countries, but the higher mysteries of the logic behind French driving habits continue to elude me. I would not lightly venture out behind the wheel of a tank into that nine o'clock maelstrom of furiously honking Citroëns and wobbling bicycles. But a chimpanzee!

"Does he know the way?" I stalled nervously.

"Of course he does, you can rely on Henri," was the reply.

The hotel commissionaire came over and also reassured me. "Don't worry, monsieur," he said. " 'E 'as been 'ere to collect guests before."

I did not dare ask whether all the previous guests were alive and well and living in sanatoria. Instead I walked up to the motorcycle. The chimpanzee looked at me blandly, raised himself, and kicked the starter. *Brrrm-brrrm, brrrm-brrrm!* He revved the engine expertly with one hairy black hand and picked his nose slowly with the other. *Brrrm-brrrrm!* I put my leg over the machine and sat down on the pillion seat tentatively, keeping some of my weight on my feet, ready to bail out at the first sign of disaster. Henri now looked straight ahead. He revved again, short crackling bursts of the two-stroke engine. I put my arms round the muscular waist of my driver and stuck my thumbs firmly into the top of his trousers.

I think it was at this stage that I began to perspire. Henri looked to his right, stopped picking his nose, revved more strongly, and then, when he saw a gap in the traffic, kicked in the gear with a practised bare foot and slipped away from the curb in a tight turn.

"Put your feet up, M. Taylor," I heard M. Godot call as he pulled out behind us into the road.

I lifted my feet onto the rests and found to my delight that we were cruising up the boulevard in a straight line at about fifteen miles an hour. Unlike the drivers of several of the vehicles on either side of us, Henri knew where he was going and how to go about it. We approached a red light. I tensed. I was definitely perspiring now. The cross-traffic was in full spate. Was it really true that chimpanzees were colour blind? This seemed a novel way of finding out.

Henri slowed down and, like the good motorcyclist he was, maintained our balance at very slow speed by weaving slowly from side to side until the lights changed. They did. *Brrrm-brrrm-br-ooom!* Henri took us smartly away with a flick of the wrist and an effortless change of gear.

The next obstacle was a traffic policeman. No problem. As Henri and I approached, the officer smiled, held up the cross-flow, and waved us on. Henri crackled past him without so much as a nod or a "bonjour."

We were getting close to the zoo but would now have to negotiate some narrow streets with several sharp corners. At the end of the boulevard we came to the first turn. I hunched over the handlebars, Henri leaned beautifully into the bend. Less accustomed to motorcycles and without the chimpanzee's perfect sense of balance, I rocked awkwardly on my seat and clutched Henri's tummy. The machine wobbled. Uncomplainingly Henri corrected the wobble. I did not dare look round to see if M. Godot was still following. Henri stared fixedly ahead, and I crouched uncomfortably behind his purposefully hunched body.

Henri took us nippily along the street, overtook a man pushing a handcart, swerved into the gutter to avoid a dog lying in the middle of the road, and then got us back on course by a smart twist of the handlebars. Two more corners, down a hill fast enough to make Henri's saucer-shaped ears flip back, and, with a turn into which he leaned over with what seemed to me more than a little flashiness,

we arrived in the zoo drive. Henri cut the revs back and
we tootled through the grounds to the ape house, where
he braked, brought the bike to a halt, and stood supporting
it with his feet while the engine ticked over.

I dismounted and walked round to face my driver,
who looked at me unblinkingly and began to pick his nose
again. It was all in a day's work for a chimp. Just a routine
pick-up, nothing to get excited about. I would have liked
to have left a small tip with my chauffeur, but I was unable
to find a banana among my small change.

I walked over to the dolphin pool. It was a beautiful
day. The overnight rain had left the air cool and fresh,
and the sunshine was streaming down on the blue-green
water. But only one dolphin cruised languidly around
where there should have been two. I felt suddenly cold.
Although dolphins in the wild are said to be able to remain
submerged for up to fifteen minutes, in captivity they
never stay down for anything like that time. When only
one blow hole broke the surface in the space of three
minutes, my fears were confirmed. The sick dolphin had
died. Kneeling down on the edge of the pool and shading
my eyes against the reflection from the water surface, I
scanned the murky depths. Sure enough, a still dark shape
lay in the shadows in the corner of the pool.

When the men arrived we got the corpse to the surface and I did a post-mortem examination. Too late I felt
the enlarged glands which bulged under the jaws and in
the throat. Cutting them open with a scalpel I saw them
to be ten times their normal size and angrily inflamed.
Mumps. This creature of the open ocean where human
viruses are unknown had fallen prey to an infection inno-
cently carried by one of the children excitedly crowding
round the pool at the end of one of the dolphin performances.

Sadly I returned to England. Perhaps I would have been unable to do anything to alter the outcome even the day before, but that's the rub. Who can say? Even now sometimes, when Shelagh asks me to change a light bulb or serves up a piece of iced gâteau, I think of that luckless animal and wonder perhaps . . . perhaps if . . . perhaps?

9 Andrew

COMING BACK FROM A TRIP to the Far East which immediately followed my New Year's trip to France, I found that
Shelagh had as usual coped brilliantly with the practice
while I was away. Nevertheless, these long trips abroad
meant that some of my clients, such as Belle Vue Zoo, were
left uncovered during my absence. Of course, the veterinarians at my old practice could stand in for me in emergencies, but their work was essentially with domestic and
farm animals, and while I could ask them to travel the
twelve miles to Manchester and Belle Vue they could not
be expected to go to the other clients that I was developing
in other parts of Britain.

It was going to be difficult to develop an exotic animal
practice single-handedly. Its very success would be self-
limiting. The more I attended to one client in one part of
the country, the more risk that I would neglect clients in
other parts. And whereas stopgap telephone advice could
hold the fort when I was in one part of Britain, it was not
easy to do this when I was travelling abroad. I got to the
point of dreading my first phone call to Shelagh when I
arrived back in the country after being overseas. What
would I hear? Some tragedy in my absence? Some client

disgruntled at my absence when faced with an emergency and resorting to disastrous self-treatment or perhaps losing the animal through waiting too long? What a way to lose clients! While I was struggling to find pygmy sperm whales in Pakistan, an orang might be dying in Manchester. And while I discussed the diseases of pangolins with veterinarians in San Diego, a crocodile in Birmingham might be in desperate need of an operation on an obstructed bowel.

Fortunately Shelagh is very good at handling the owners of small exotic pets. Over the years she has gained a wide knowledge of animal medicine and first-aid care. She can deal with the overwrought owners of a dying senile hamster or an iguana with an abscess on its leg with consummate finesse. Her deep love of all animals comes across, and her willingness to take the time to discuss the facts of the case make her extremely effective. She doesn't play at being a vet, doesn't institute courses of injections or prescribe antibiotics. Her forte is in reassuring the owner, instructing in good nursing care, and starting simple emergency measures if required. She makes notes, and when I am away I ring up at least once a day to discuss any minor cases which await my return. She will go through the list of lizards, monkeys, parrots, and the like which she has dealt with, and we will discuss what further action is necessary.

Nevertheless, the problem of one man trying to be in two places at the same time became increasingly acute as my work abroad expanded. I obviously needed a partner, and luckily for me the perfect man was right at hand.

Andrew Greenwood first appeared on the scene after I had been working at Flamingo Park for several months. He was still a student at Cambridge and had been introduced to me by a vet who had once been my assistant in general practice and with whom Andrew had been gaining experience by "seeing practice" during the vacations. The vet had phoned me and asked me if I would care to let this young chap, who had a brilliant academic record and an intense interest in zoo animal matters, spend some time with me at Flamingo Park.

I enjoy teaching and have always been more than willing to accept as many students as I could in this way. The experience is an essential part of a vet's training, and I had myself profited immensely by it when I was a student. But as I moved increasingly into purely zoo practice it had become far less easy to organize. It isn't possible for a student to accompany me on my travels abroad for the obvious reason of expense, and in some areas of work with wild species the presence of unqualified or inexperienced personnel can be downright dangerous; one student attending a case with me at Dudley Zoo, for example, had had his spectacles snatched from him and destroyed by a chimpanzee.

I vividly remember another time when a second student, a girl, accompanied me to Belle Vue Zoo, where we examined from a distance of about twenty feet an obstreperous bull oryx which was displaying certain peculiarities of gait. The two of us stood just inside the door of the paddock with the head keeper and discussed the possible reasons for the animal's developing lameness. Suddenly, without any warning and with the agility and speed for which the creature is noted, it spun towards us, lowered its black sabre-like horns towards our torsos, and charged full pelt.

Pure reflex action propelled us back in blind panic. One of us, who knows who, wrenched the door open, and we tumbled through headlong and crashed it to behind us. As I struggled to shoot home the bolt I had a vivid recollection of how I had once seen the hard horns of an oryx packed in a wooden crate thrust through four inches of timber as if it were butter.

As we gathered ourselves together on the safe side of the door, we realized that we were two instead of three. The head keeper and I stared at one another in horror. The girl student had been left inside with the oryx! It was sickeningly plain to both of us that our alacrity had far exceeded our gallantry. Perhaps even then she was impaled against the other side of the door like a kebab.

I regret to say that our cowardice still knew no bounds. Instead of bravely flinging open the door and charging in to the rescue, we unbolted it and cautiously opened it a crack. I squinted through it anxiously, and the girl's calm face stared placidly back. Shamefacedly we let her out. The kebab was definitely unskewered and appeared remarkably unruffled. We muttered our apologies wretchedly. "Oh, don't worry about that," she said brightly, all aglow at having Done Some Real Zoo Work for the first time. "He was rather a sweet old dear, swerved away at the last moment and never so much as brushed my dress."

Yes, there can be problems in having students seeing practice in the context of a zoo. However, I agreed to let Andrew get some experience with me. For one thing he had a car and assured me that he had enough cash for any travelling that might be involved. For another, there was simply no way of getting rid of him. A thoughtful and extraordinarily laconic Yorkshireman with a public-school education, he was relentless in his search for knowledge. Like Brer Rabbit he used to say nothin' but would simply turn up and quietly participate in anything that was going on. If I forgot to inform him that an operation was to take place or that I was going to drain the whale pool for blood

sampling at two o'clock in the morning or load some
elephants for transport on a Saturday evening, somehow
he would find out through the bush telegraph and turn up.
He never got in the way but was always ready to lend a
hand if asked. Most of all I noticed that he was an avid
pursuer of his own lines of interest and inquiry. If there
was any minute quantity of blood left over in the bottles
after I had taken all I needed for my examinations he
would be off with them to study on his own, and when I
had completed an operation or a necropsy he would pick
meticulously over any remains of diseased tissue that I had
removed, or the scattered debris of the carcass.

Our first meeting at Flamingo Park might not have
seemed very auspicious. Andrew arrived bright-eyed and
bushy-tailed, with casebook and camera in hand, all set to
begin an intensive few weeks of zoo vet practice, only to
find that half an hour later I had to dash off to catch a
plane for Copenhagen. When I got back to Flamingo Park
ten days had passed and I had forgotten all about him. But
he was still there, just as if I had only been away ten minutes, and what was more I found that he had not wasted
his time but had occupied himself in getting useful background knowledge in the way a zoo park functions.

During his final years at university Andrew stuck to
me like a limpet. His interest in zoo work blazed unabat-
edly and he didn't seem to be seduced in any way by the
temptations of a more orthodox career with farm animals,
in small animal practice, or in research. He kept close tabs
on what I was doing, taking ever more bits of material
from my cases when I had finished with them for his own
investigations. When he qualified he decided to take a
Royal Navy grant to study the brain of diving mammals.
We never discussed a future together, but looking back it
seems as if that were a tacit assumption. My work was

developing an increasing emphasis on the problems of marine animals, and Andrew's work as a post-graduate student in the department of Professor Richard Harrison, one of the world's leading authorities on whales and dolphins, would fit neatly into place. We complemented one another in our special areas of interest and in everything else we did, as if we were developing our lives jointly to some invisible plan. While Andrew was concentrating on research, on academic work contacts with Establishment zoologists, on falcons and wildfowl, papers at learned societies, and a working knowledge of French and Russian, I was out in the field knocking out, opening up, stitching, injecting, and coming eyeball to eyeball with land and sea mammals, hobnobbing with the down-market impresarios of commercial zoo parks and circuses, packaging veterinary and zoological material for television and the media, and learning Spanish and Chinese as a hobby. The beauty of having Andrew stay at Cambridge on the diving work was that he was freely available to stand in for me whenever I was called out of the country.

Of course it was not easy to get clients to accept new assistants or substitutes, particularly in my line. The whole business is highly personalized, since it requires special knowledge and the patients are usually very valuable. As a young vet starting work on the bleak moorland farms around my home, I'd met plenty of initial resistance from cantankerous farmers who'd say, "I've nought against you, son, but I don't want you practising on one of my cows!" Andrew had to go through a bit of the same in a zoo context. As I had done years before, he cut his teeth on some of the day-to-day problems at Belle Vue. There Shelagh, with the innumerable tips and common sense about animals that she'd amassed since we had got married, could back him up while I was away.

I sent him on his first mission to Windsor Safari Park, a zoo set on a hillside facing ancient Windsor Castle in the historic town 30 miles outside London, to tranquillize a group of timid wallabies that were being brought in. Just the stress brought on in these creatures by grabbing hold of them can be enough to give them fatal heart attacks. All survived. While I was away in Germany treating some beluga whales, Shelagh dispatched him to deal with a pair of dying leopards at a circus in the Midlands. If I'd known I would have fretted about how he was going to gain access to one of the most suspicious and xenophobic troupes in the country, and how, if he did get in, he would tackle anaesthetizing and then reviving the highly dangerous big cats in the mean and unequipped wagon of the travelling menagerie. I need not have worried. All went perfectly.

No doubt it was unreasonable to develop, as I had done, the conviction that all the different zoo animals with which I had built up a relationship in health and sickness over a number of years were in safe hands only if I was on the scene, and that I had some sort of exclusive control over their fortunes. However, I am still convinced that animals are affected by the mood and will and mental attitude of the humans caring for them. Drugs and instruments are not everything. On numerous occasions I have demonstrated, at least to myself, that when I am in a buoyant, thrusting, optimistic frame of mind my cases tend to progress well, whereas if I am depressed or preoccupied I seem to lose a psychic element of influence for which medicines and surgery alone cannot always compensate. All this is bound up with the fact that almost all my patients are old friends. And even if I've never seen a particular animal before, I feel I know it well because others of the same species are my friends.

Nonetheless, whether I liked it or not Andrew happily

took over my cases while I was abroad and got on with
diagnosing, treating, and curing his first animal illnesses.
There turned out to be few grumbles from my clients,
and those few were sometimes of a surprising kind. One
dolphin owner complained bitterly about Andrew's technique in necropsying one of his animals. "He took poor old
Flipper literally to pieces! Reduced him to a thousand
and one little bits! Minced up in a way I'm sure you would
never have done, Dr. Taylor." Andrew as usual had been
extremely thorough in making his post-mortem examination; every portion of every organ had been minutely
examined and, where suspicious, sampled, bottled, and
labelled. The study of dead animals causes them no suffering and leads to new hope and benefit for the living. Of
course necropsies are hardly aesthetic affairs, though they
can be immensely elegant and fascinating. It wasn't easy
trying to explain to the dolphin owner that Flipper as a
plastic sack full of little bits was an example of veterinary
thoroughness and responsibility of a much higher standard
than the more reverential and tidy "unzip down the middle,
have a look in, and if the cause of death doesn't jump out
at you, sew up again" post-mortems that some people are
satisfied by.

As I became busier and Andrew did more work for
me I noticed other things. More and more people would
arrive at the house with small exotic birds: finches and
canaries, parakeets and humming-birds. There were also
old ladies who had rescued common sparrows and black-
birds, all of which Andrew would attend to meticulously.
He adores birds, whereas somehow they fail to fire my
imagination. Another thing I noticed was that, just as Andrew had attached himself to me when he was a student,
now he was beginning to attract disciples exhibiting the
same leech-like qualities. Sometimes when there was a

particularly important operation or an unusual case I would ask Andrew to accompany me, and his apprentices would tag along too. It got to the point that zoo visits were conducted by a chain of masters and pupils, with me as the old guru at one end trailed by Andrew and his acolytes in a descending order of age and experience down to a first-year veterinary student with an unquenchable thirst for beer. It cost me a fortune to refresh my little band at the local hostelry after a day's work.

At last the point came, without any preliminary discussion, when Andrew and I decided to go into partnership. We had just finished operating on a baboon with an ingrowing wisdom tooth one day when I said, "Why don't we go and see a solicitor and draw up an agreement as fifty-fifty partners?"

"Good idea," replied Andrew, with typical brevity. He gave a month's notice to the Navy and it was done. From now on we could expand everything together. I was very pleased.

After the partnership was formed we slipped into the relaxed and easy working relationship which has persisted to this day. While I roam about the south of England Andrew looks after matters in the north, or vice versa, and we try to take the longer trips abroad alternately so that each of us can spend some time at home. Sometimes it happens that both of us are out of Britain at the same time, and then Shelagh has to hold the fort. I don't think she likes it very much, and it is true that on such occasions animals on our home patch are vulnerable, although we make a point of telephoning her at a regular hour each day. At least one of us is always within striking distance of an airport in Europe and able to fly back if a serious emergency should arise. Shelagh stays on tenterhooks because she has the job of identifying exactly what are the serious emergencies, but through good luck and her excellent management we have so far never had anything that needed urgent attention go neglected, nor has she ever dragged us back for something that proved to be a false alarm.

At first it seemed that there might only be about one and a third men's work for the two of us to do, and we would often spend hours sitting in the little office at my home, one on each side of the battered old partners' desk that we'd acquired, reading about zoo animals or hammering out a common approach to their health problems. I can't remember our ever having an argument, although our styles are not at all alike. I'm sure Andrew looked down his nose a bit at some of the gimmicky things I would go along with for the press. For instance, I was filmed for television with an orang-utan adult who had had some teeth extracted; the sleeping ape was shown reclining in a dental chair with its head bound with an old-fashioned pad and bandage. On the other hand, I used to raise my eyebrows but say nothing when presented with large bills for the books Andrew purchased regularly for our library. Expensive and narrowly specialized tomes about birds or amphibians were hardly likely to be profit-yielding investments in the monetary sense.

Our periods of relative underemployment also enabled us to accompany one another on visits to cases from time to time. The client got two veterinarians for the price of one, and we got a chance to compare notes and learn together. It also meant that, both of us being keen trenchermen, we could dine out around Britain and improve our appreciation of wine along with our scientific deliberations.

Quiet and studious as he was, Andrew was nonetheless attractive to the girls, and I began to find an increasing number of calls for routine examinations and blood samplings of animals on the continent where he was specifically requested. A small coterie of travelling shows, dolphinaria, and circuses, usually with pretty unmarried lady presenters and trainers, increasingly asked for Dr. Greenwood to be sent out. Requests increased for him to telephone Fifi or Lulu in person with advice on worming the sea-lions or telling the age of a crocodile or how many beans make five. I must admit that at one stage I wondered whether some artful beauty might hook him and he'd end up as travelling medical man with some French circus or other. But Andrew appeared quite impervious. Off he would go to Switzerland or Germany or wherever it was, steadfastly treat his animals, and sort out the problems. Then, for he has a remarkable liver, he would drink them under the table when they entertained him in the evening and return home the following day full of enthusiasm about the case he had seen and the samples he had brought back and definitely unsnared. "He takes his work very seriously, doesn't he?" was the rueful remark of all the young ladies in question whenever they had to put up with my presence.

Only once did I hear of Andrew letting his hair down, when he went to treat some animals for the high-class Gasser's dolphin show in Switzerland. After a hard day catching, blood-sampling, and vaccinating a group of dolphins, Andrew went with Conny Gasser, a good friend of ours, and some of the staff to a little *weinstube* famed for its home-made pear liqueur. The beverage must have possessed remarkable properties, for I was amazed to hear how Andrew had delighted the assembled company by listening through his stethoscope, for what I know not, to the buttocks of a buxom Swiss barmaid.

Eventually Andrew got married to Linda, a girl from Leeds and a childhood sweetheart. In our work even weddings aren't sacrosanct. First I was called out of the ceremony to take a call from Majorca about an injured sea-lion, and then at the end of the wedding reception there was an urgent message from Germany about two sick dolphins. I was already scheduled to go to Holland, so I had to ask the happy pair if they minded changing their plans and making it a working honeymoon in Berlin. Both of them agreed, and their married life began by struggling in the bottom of a smelly, partly drained pool to pass stomach tubes down the throats of the two sick animals.

When they got back from Berlin we had another surprise in store for them: a week's trip for Andrew, alone, to Spain! When he came back from that would he go for a couple of weeks to Israel and then make a tour of India, looking at every white tiger in that country, returning by way of Egypt to do a couple of days' work there? In the end Andrew spent only three and a half days at home with Linda during their first eight weeks of nuptial bliss.

One of the rare occasions when Andrew and I travelled together abroad concerned camels. Camels are fascinating animals, tough, uncomplaining about work, and beautifully and functionally built, but their spit seems to have an affinity for suede leather and can never be removed, as I discovered when, clad in an expensive and much prized suede jacket but unprotected by an overall, I examined my first camel.

I knew as we all do that camels spit, but I did not realize what little it takes to make them do it. Camels will spit at the slightest provocation, real or imagined; they will spit pre-emptively to start trouble or defensively when one merely looks at them in the wrong way. What is more, camel spit is a bottomless well of smelly, green, partly digested stomach contents that is sprayed as a broadside or aimed in a single noxious blob of flying soup. This makes examining camels something of a specialized art. Putting an old jacket over the camel's head is said to help, but I have known a wily beast to spit accurately down the sleeves of the garment.

Camels can also kick in any direction with any or all of their legs, and they try to heighten the effect of spitting by making awful gurgling noises and extruding a heaving pink sausage, part of the lining of the mouth, from between yellow teeth. Finally, they can bite very severely and with purpose. Moses, a magnificent but cantankerous male Bactrian camel at Manchester, is one of the most dangerous zoo animals I know. He fractured the skull and broke both arms and the thigh of a kindly old man who, without permission, went into the camel pen to stroke him.

Camels may build up a pressure cooker of resentment towards human beings until the lid suddenly blows off and they go berserk. In Asia when a camel gets to this high pitch of bottled-up tension the camel driver senses the brooding trouble and takes off his coat and gives it to the animal. Then, rather like Japanese workers who are provided with special rooms where they can work off their frustrations and resentments by beating up models of their executives, the camel gives the garment hell, jumping on it, ripping it, biting it, tearing it to pieces. When the camel feels that it has blown its top enough, man and animal can live together in harmony again.

Andrew and I had ample opportunity to study the contrariness of the species at close quarters when we went twice in the same day from Manchester to Prague to pick up a consignment of Bactrian camels for Marwell Zoo near Winchester. Andrew selected the beefiest of his disciples to come along with us. We might well need some extra muscle. The camels were from Asian Russia, semi-wild and grumpy. Some had vicious rope halters running tightly round their heads and through holes bored in their ears. They had been branded on the cheeks with hot irons months or years before and had been fitted with the halters when quite small. As the camels had grown the halters had cut deep into the flesh and in some places had disappeared completely beneath the skin. Before loading in Prague our first job was to cut off these evil devices, but even so it was too late for one poor creature. The dirty rope sawing away at its head had introduced tetanus germs into the body and it was showing the first symptoms of lockjaw, a terrible disease to witness. At least when we got it back to Manchester we were able to give it treatment and relieve the agonizing muscular spasms, but the unfortunate animal died.

Everything went well with the loading at Prague. A Communist soldier stood guard outside the aircraft's lavatory door to ensure that no one stowed away in there, while the poor veterinary surgeon from Prague Zoo who had handed the animals over to us was not allowed to set foot inside the cargo hold or cabin at all. He would dearly have liked to see his charges settled down in the plane, but the authorities were not taking any chances that he might somehow disappear among the grunting, shuffling crowd of Bactrians. Instead, we gave him a bottle of whisky and some bottles of a superb new zoo animal anaesthetic, and he gave us in exchange some Czech aerosols for treating skin diseases.

The camels behaved themselves perfectly. Once aboard the aircraft almost all of them sat quietly down, and we did not need to use a single dose of sedative. The flight back to Manchester was uneventful, with not so much as a peep out of the animals, and we landed easily at Ringway Airport, where transport and lots of keepers from the zoo were waiting to help us unload.

While I arranged the disposition of our troops, An-

drew did a masterly job of distracting the attention of the
waiting government veterinary officer by engaging him in
conversation. As the aircraft's unloading doors were
opened we had seen a quantity of straw, theoretically contaminated because these were foreign animals coming into
quarantine, fall out of the fuselage, get picked up by the
wind, and disperse over the airfield. Such things were
taboo, and although there wasn't much one could do about
it the government man could have caused trouble. Andrew
saw that the vet had not spotted the straw falling from the
plane and manoeuvred the fellow around by talking almost
nose to nose with him until the errant shreds of bedding
had whisked out of sight.

By this time all the camels were sitting down and relaxing. They were superb air travellers. Now we had to
get them onto their feet to walk them down the ramp into
the special fly-screened quarantine van that would take
them to the zoo. Camels and their relatives, the llamas,
alpacas, and vicuñas, are easily offended. They sit down
for a variety of reasons, such as annoyance, disgust, bore-
dom, fright, or just to be uncooperative. Sometimes, of
course, they sit down for the pleasure of it. When sitting
down they may insist on rising for the same reasons.
The general rule is that they will do the exact opposite
of what the humans round them want them to do. This was
a typical case: The entire cargo decided, as one camel, not
to get to its feet. Presumably they felt that they had done
us enough favours that day in allowing themselves to be
loaded so easily and then transported across Europe and
that now it was time for them to give us a bit of stick.

We tried shouting, slapping, lifting tails, blowing down
ears, and prodding with a stick. Nothing worked. Camel
spittle began to fly around. Not one solitary camel was
prepared to budge. They sat quietly resting on their bris-

kets as if bolted to the floor. In the end they won. Each
one had to be lifted and carried bodily down to the van
with the men bending and linking hands with one another
beneath the chests, bellies, and groins of the beasts to form
a sweating, straining human sling. It breaks the backs of
five or six men to pick up a mature camel in this way, and
we had fifteen on board and another fifteen in the second
consignment waiting in Prague.

At last it was done. We flew back to Czechoslovakia
and collected the rest. Again they travelled perfectly but,
once they had landed at Manchester, became completely
unco-operative and had to be carried out like the first
bunch. It made the sweating keepers curse when some
strapping great bull, which had just insisted on being borne
out like a pitiful stretcher case, stood up voluntarily when
deposited in the quarantine van and projected a gurgling
stream of stomach contents at his erstwhile bearers.

Andrew's dogged fascination with the minutiae of
necropsy examinations, and his collecting of sundry anatomical bits and pieces with which he carries on long after
I've got my provisional diagnosis of cause of death and
called it a day, is as pronounced now as when I first met
him. He collects these shreds and snippets of organs and
tissues not only for himself but also for a growing number of friends and colleagues, and at each post-mortem he
draws up a sort of bizarre gift list, a sharing of the spoils
in the war against disease. To him, a dead porpoise or
hyena means one kidney for Dr. A in London, who spe-
cializes in renal disease; the other kidney for Dr. B in Los
Angeles, who has requested such an item for a research
project in immunology; both testes or ovaries for Professor
C in Cambridge, who, maybe, will be able to age the dead
animal precisely or trace its past breeding activity; and a

one-inch square of skin for the British Museum, which will add it to their collection of reference specimens in the natural history department.

His zeal for things anatomical paid off during our post-mortem on a whale which died after a long illness in Italy. We had both flown down several times before to advise on the medical treatment of the case, which presented one marked and central symptom, a precipitate, persistent, and uncheckable fall in the blood's white cell count. Something was knocking out the sources of production of these necessary cells in the bone marrow. We could find no source of serious infection or toxin which might be doing this, and our efforts to boost white cell production by drugs met no success. When the animal died we both went out for the necropsy.

The whale had been insured by the owner for many thousands of dollars, and to make a claim would require a veterinary certificate. This would have to be issued, we were told, by an Italian vet. The owner arranged for the local dog and cat veterinarian to attend and issue the necessary document. Andrew and I did the examination, a business that took many hours in a creature that was nearly twenty feet long. The Italian veterinarian hovered about us, clucking about this and that and prating on to all the bystanders about the internal organs of a species with which he was utterly unfamiliar. On and on we cut, bloody from head to toe, standing in our underpants within the gargantuan carcass itself. Andrew meticulously opened every little lymph gland and every inch of the yards of intestine. Nothing seemed wrong. No abscesses, no areas of dead or inflamed tissue, no evidence of poisons, no malignancies or foreign bodies.

By the end of the day we came to the heart. The Italian veterinarian was still there, but he was growing increasingly testy. He seemed to feel we should have produced something satisfyingly horrendous hours ago if we knew what we were about. When Andrew opened the pericardium, the membrane around the heart, a small but abnormal amount of blood-tinged fluid ran out. It was the only unusual thing we had come across, although it was not sufficient in itself to account in any way for symptoms seen and certainly not for the fatal outcome.

"*Ecco!*" cried the Italian veterinarian with much flailing of his arms when he saw the trickle of liquid. "I have found it! A heart attack. The whale died from a heart attack without doubt!" Producing his pen, he proceeded to make out a health certificate. "I have found it, I have found it," he repeated, and then having handed over the piece of paper he advised everyone to go home.

During all this I told Andrew to say nothing. We saw no reason why the owner should not get his insurance money. No negligence had been involved, that was certain. But we had failed to find anything that explained the case. The Italian vet, though in error, had at least given them something to hang their hats on. As everyone cleaned up and prepared to leave, I considered letting the cause of death remain a mystery until the bacteriological and virus examination of our samples was made. That might reveal something.

Andrew, however, had no such intention; he announced that he was going to ferret away at the carcass all night long if necessary. First, however, he needed a short rest, so he stuck his scalpel into a handy place, which happened to be the skin on the whale's back.

As he did so, we heard a faint but most remarkable sound: a brief hissing noise as the blade pierced the blubber. Instantaneously we both looked at one another. There was no need to say anything; we had heard, rather than seen, the first clue. "Not a word until our Italian friend has driven off in his car," I murmured to Andrew through clenched teeth. "Let's come back later when everyone has gone home."

We did. Near midnight, we recommenced our examination by torchlight like a couple of grave robbers. Andrew stripped off the skin and blubber of the back of the whale around the area where he had stuck in the scalpel. Underneath in the giant lumbar muscles that power the drive of the tail flukes, we saw a black, gas-pocketed area of tissue about as big as a man's hand. The hissing noise had been made by escaping gas produced by the feeding of a special class of bacteria which kill by producing chemical toxins rather than by invading the body extensively themselves. It was the so-called gas gangrene, the scourge of wounded soldiers in the trenches of World War I.

Andrew investigated the tissues for several hours, and gradually the likely origin of this unusual infection, which had been hidden beneath tight layers of skin and blubber, became clear. Repeated injections in the back (the whale had received more than one hundred shots over the space of a week or two) had devitalized the tissues and weakened their resistance in the local area. Then, possibly through faulty sterilization of needles or because air spores just happened to land on a needle hole, the bacterium had found an opportunity to settle into a cosy, airless abode where it could go about its secret and deadly business.

We decided to have a quiet word with the trainer who had been in charge of the whale-injecting, a conscientious chap who, we considered, had been unlucky rather than careless. But rightly or wrongly we let sleeping dogs lie as far as other folk were concerned, speaking neither to the Italian veterinarian nor to the owner. It was better that the whale remain on their records as "Heart attack."

10 The Big Knockout

SOME PROFESSIONS HAVE their particularly acute and awesome moments, when one man in naked isolation holds the total responsibility for precipitating a great event. So it must be for the diamond cutter who, after months of carefully studying and measuring a stone of great value, finally raises his arm to strike the first blow that will either cleave it brilliantly or mar it irreparably. The engineer who must demolish a smokestack, having calculated the exact strength and disposition of explosives needed, placed his charges carefully, and worked out where the rubble will fall, must inevitably take the detonator handle into his grasp and with one deliberate movement initiate either an ordered dissolution or complete chaos.

In my work such moments are associated with the times when it becomes imperative to knock out one of the great land mammals, to lay low a living, breathing, sentient ton or two of muscle and bone and sinew. The great beast has to be rendered peacefully inert for a measured space of time, quickly enough to avoid any halfway stage of panic-stricken delirium or dizziness, and yet not so quickly that the head of the animal, dropping from the height of a first-storey window, cracks like an egg on the ground below.

My moment of truth is when I have delivered by dart
or hypodermic syringe a full knockout dose of anaesthetic
to a standing adult giraffe or elephant. When I hear the
pop of the small explosive charge inside the dart as it goes
home or feel my thumb come to a stop as the last drop of
liquid is expressed from the syringe, a strange coolness
begins to circulate in my veins. The animal before me and
myself are the sole living things in a silent black universe;
we are linked by an invisible umbilical cord. It is the most
stunning experience in my life. The injection is a *fait ac-
compli,* and now, carrying the little piece of me with it,
it travels unseen yet omnipotent first through the capil-
laries, then through the veins that feed the heart, out to
cascade through the lungs, and once more back to the
heart, and then begins the steep climb up the arteries leading through the neck towards the brain. I wait during the
long icy seconds for the drug to arrive at the brain cells,
until the eyes suddenly glaze, the great legs turn limp, and
with a sigh the towering creature comes down to my size,
gently received by a layer of straw. But I am the victor
only if the heart is beating soundly and the lungs continue
gently to breathe.

And shortly thereafter, I have to face a second moment of truth, to spin the film backwards and put the
giant back up where it came from by bringing it out of the
anaesthetic and back into the world again, alert and un-
frightened, without pain or panic. Each operation then on
these big animals has these two climactic points when I
have the very essence of the life force of the biggest,
wildest, strongest, strangest beasts in the palm of my
hand.

When I first started out in general practice in the late
fifties, I was severely handicapped in treating zoo ani-

mals by the fact that there existed neither an effective, well-tolerated anaesthetic for a vast range of species with differing anatomies and physiological functions, nor a good means of administering it. Of course we had the barbiturates, which worked well if injected into a vein, but how does one persuade a pain-racked rhino to stand still while you raise its jugular with the pressure of one thumb and squeeze in an intravenous needle with the other? New gases such as halothane were superseding ether and chloroform, but what persuades a sea-lion to inhale the soporific vapour in the face mask when, as an accomplished deep-sea diver, it is used to holding its breath for ten minutes at a time? Drugs which in capsule or tablet form bring speedy oblivion to a human with an empty stomach tended to get lost in the hundredweights of digesting food and churning liquid inside a hippo's or an elephant's stomach. Or they produced bizarre responses, as when I tried one reliable human tranquillizer by mouth on bison. Instead of making the animals calm and sleepy, it whipped them into an amazing state of sexual frenzy, transforming even the most decrepit old males into bellowing satyrs which dashed about mounting every female they could lay their hooves on.

The lack of an effective anaesthetic at that time was brought home sharply to me when I was called to Belle Vue Zoo to examine Mary, an Indian elephant. One of the zoo's oldest inhabitants, she had been suffering from increasingly severe attacks of toothache. Elephants have a peculiar tooth arrangement with a system of continual replacement of the grinding molars throughout their lifetime. The teeth develop from buds at one end of a groove in the jaw, move forward into use as they grow, and then fall out, to be replaced by others coming along the groove behind them. This process sometimes hits snags. A tooth jams instead of falling out cleanly and the animal shows all the signs of tenderness and irritation in the mouth that humans would associate with an impacted wisdom tooth.

Mary's problem was one stage worse than this: She had developed an abscess at the base of a tooth root in the lower jaw. The abscess enlarged and caused severe pain within the unyielding confines of the bony jaw. Mary became nervous and grumpy. She ate little other than soft over-ripe bananas. She drooled saliva more than usual and would open her mouth for inspection only with great reluctance.

At my first examination I asked the keeper to persuade Mary to open her mouth. Eventually, after lots of soothing talk, I could put my hand inside. Feeling about in an elephant's mouth is not the least hazardous of veterinary procedures. There is not much room, and it is easy to find one's fingers being pushed by the strong muscular tongue between the grinding surfaces of the teeth, a most excruciating experience. When I tapped the infected molar with the back of my knuckle, Mary pulled back, beat me lustily about the head with her trunk, and screeched like a pig. With a root abscess in other animals, one would extract the tooth and all would be well. But in an elephant it was quite a different matter. The tooth in question was firmly embedded in the jaw and, like all elephant teeth, had multiple curved roots which swept deep down into the jawbone and interwove intricately with the bony tissue around them. Pulling, even with giant forceps, was out of the question and so was elevating, the flicking out of a tooth by means of a lever-like instrument. I decided to try medical treatment instead, to destroy the abscess by injections of antibiotics and to relieve pain by injectable analgesics.

The snag with this course is that the trouble tends to flare up again some weeks or months later. Sure enough, the injections produced a rapid disappearance of all symptoms and within a day Mary was once more her own amenable self. Two or three weeks later, however, the zoo rang up to say that Mary was beginning to show the same symptoms again, but this time the pain was so bad that she was banging her head against the wall. I drove down at once to Manchester and, sure enough, a very forlorn Mary once again had an abscess under the same tooth. The drug injections quickly put matters right and the following day the elephant had stopped the head-banging.

Over the next six months Mary had four more attacks of toothache involving the same tooth root, and each attack was more severe and lasted longer than the one before. The head-banging became the principal symptom. Mary would stand for hours close to the wall of the elephant house, deliberately rocking on her ankles and crashing the affected side of her head against the brickwork with a regular, dull, horrible thud that could be heard two hundred yards away. She had knocked the paint off a large area of the wall and loosened the pointing between the bricks.

The fourth attack was the worst. Mary refused all food but stood night and day against the wall, seeking to counter the aching focus in her jaw by temporarily distracting the throbbing nerves as one ton of head jarred into the brickwork. It was terrible to listen to and unpleasant to watch; she was bruising and cutting the skin on the side of her face and becoming ill-tempered and unpredictable. What was more, the wall was beginning to bulge outwards, many bricks were loose, and the zoo director feared that the structure of the building was now at serious risk. We had to do something more positive. The tooth causing all the trouble would have to come out.

It was clear that the only way to remove the offending

molar was to perform a major operation on the jaw. The gum along the side of the tooth root would have to be flapped up and the thick covering plate of bone chipped away, and then the tooth with its roots intact could be teased, cajoled, and manoeuvred sideways out of the jaw. This would mean a long period under general anaesthetic; a shot of local as performed by the dentist, or even a nerve block, the numbing of the nerve to the tooth by surrounding it with local anaesthetic at some point on its path back towards the brain, would not be feasible. The area of tissue involved was too large and complicated and the animal was in far too agitated a state. Anyway, it would be impossible to do the necessary work unless she was lying down with her head still.

Because no really suitable general anaesthetic was available, major operations on elephants had rarely been performed. Local anaesthetic was used for minor matters, but otherwise it had been a question of tying the poor creature down with chains and hobbles and using the crudest of methods. Giving chloroform or ether was virtually impossible; barbiturates had to be given intravenously in ridiculously large doses, had a nasty knack of damaging adjacent veins and tissues, and depressed breathing seriously; while chloral hydrate, the old standby of horse practitioners, was so disgustingly bitter when given in water that an animal would need to be stopped from drinking for three or four days before it would accept the doctored liquid. I decided to look into the possibility of injecting a new and promising drug which I had been using for two or three years on other exotic creatures.

Giving Mary a stiff dose of pain-killer and antibiotics to relieve the situation, I announced that we would operate on her the following day and that suitable preparations should be made. Then I went home to consider the matter further.

The new drug, phencyclidine, had been the first important breakthrough in modern zoo animal anaesthesia. It was highly concentrated, formed a stable solution which had no annoying tendency to go off, and was effective when given either by injection under the skin, by mouth, or in a flying dart. Its taste was not too bitter, so that when used to spike the fruit drinks or milk of those discerning and wide-awake customers, the great apes, it usually went down unnoticed.

There were disadvantages, too. The dose was calculated on body weight, and once it was administered there was no way of neutralizing its effects, which wore off gradually over a number of hours. Some animals such as polar bears were easily overdosed with the stuff; I had noticed how little phencyclidine they needed to knock them flat out compared with brown or Himalayan black bears. Wolves, the first animals on which I had ever used the chemical and the tranquillizing gun, frequently developed alarming convulsions when unconscious under phencyclidine. The drug had proved to be unsuitable for horses, and I had discovered to my dismay that it had serious untoward effects in zebras; instead of anaesthetizing an animal which had broken out of its pen and could only be dosed by means of a flying dart containing phencyclidine, the drug produced an alarming degree of excitement and distress which persisted for hours. But in monkeys and apes, the big cats, and some other carnivores it was superb. We never saw any signs of the long-lasting sexual stimulant effects or burning sensations of the fingertips and toes which humans treated with the drug had reported, although big cats under phencyclidine anaesthesia do regularly extend and contract their claws. (If you look carefully at a Daktari or Tarzan film on television when our hero stands at the side of a "dying" or "sleeping" leopard or tiger, you will often notice this characteristic behaviour, a sure sign that the studio veterinarian has used phencyclidine.)

For Mary's operation, phencyclidine was the best drug I had at the time. Checking that evening through my library, I found one or two reports of its previous use on elephants, but details were scanty. What was suitable as an experimental dose in the African bush where elephants were plentiful was not necessarily right for Mary, a valuable and much-loved animal in a city zoo in the industrial north of England. I had to get the dose right.

Another problem was estimating the weight of an animal such as Mary. My usual practice is to walk the animal or take it in a lorry to a public weigh-bridge, but the toothache had made Mary crotchety and unco-operative and I could not risk taking her out of the elephant house. If an animal cannot actually be weighed, I take the average of three estimates made by myself and two other people accustomed to working with animals; with this I calculated a dose for Mary for the following morning. Certain nagging problems remained. How long would the anaesthetic last and what would be the cumulative effect of any further doses once she was down? What awkward physiological changes would several hours' unconsciousness produce in the ponderous creature? How was I to ensure that she went down with her bad tooth uppermost? It is not easy to turn a four-and-a-half-ton elephant when she is collapsed unconscious like a great pile of rock.

The next morning I was up early. My first call was to the local ironmongers. Dental instruments for human or ordinary veterinary use are far too puny for the granite-hard teeth of an elephant and the thick, resilient bone in which they are embedded. What I needed was a set of high-quality, all-metal masonry chisels. The ironmonger produced exactly what I wanted, a set of tough tungsten-edged tools specially intended for punching holes in hard stone. When I explained what they were for, the shop-keeper said he would sell them to me at tradesman's price. "After all," he said, "you're using them for your trade, I suppose. Never thought I'd find myself selling surgical instruments!"

At the zoo I found Mary suffering considerably from the diseased tooth. The pain-killing drug had worn off and she was in a black mood. As I entered her quarters she glowered down at me and shuffled agitatedly around, whisking and flailing her trunk. It was going to be difficult keeping her still enough even for the normally simple under-skin injection of phencyclidine. I decided to leave all the instruments outside until she was anaesthetized. How she would go down and whether, during the few seconds that the anaesthetic first affected her brain cells, she would feel dizzy and become alarmed, I did not know. But I remembered having cases of horses run amok during the first stages of barbiturate dosage, with disastrous effects on the surrounding and carefully sterilized equip-ment, and I was not taking any chances.

Matt Kelly, the head keeper, solved the problem of persuading Mary to stand still for a second or two while I gave her the dope. Mary had one great weakness—an unbridled appetite for custard pies, the open, nutmeg-sprinkled, Lancashire variety. Even though the toothache had quenched her desire for more conventional foods, Matt guessed that she would still be unable to resist these delicacies, and he sent up to the zoo restaurant for some. Sure enough, when a keeper appeared with a box full of the newly baked golden pastries, the demeanour of the miserable animal immediately changed. Her black mood becoming at least charcoal grey, she stopped roaming about irritably and proceeded with obvious enjoyment to roll the custards one after another into her mouth, carefully avoiding the offending left side of her jaw.

While she was thus engaged I slapped three times on her rump with the flat of my hand and then, when she was accustomed to the contact, slapped her again with equal force but this time with a three-inch needle held between my fingers. She did not feel a thing as I connected the syringe full of anaesthetic to the needle and pressed the plunger. It was in. I had begun the general anaesthesia of my first elephant.

Mary continued to consume the last of the custard pies, still standing calmly as we silently watched her. The elephant's soft munching was the only sound to be heard. Now I was going to be faced with the answers to the questions with which my mind was racing. What was the effect of the drug going to be? Was my dose adequate or perhaps even too large? Had my needle squirted it deep into a layer of fat where its absorption would be greatly delayed and the effect minimized?

A minute passed. Mary cleared the last flakes of pie pastry from her lips and looked at Matt for more. No signs of grogginess. At what time should I consider giving another dose? I wondered, clenching my fists. How would a second injection act in relation to the first? What would the cumulative effects be? Suppose the first effects on Mary were indeed to make her feel dizzy and alarmed? What if she ran amok while still sufficiently conscious to stay on her feet? For a moment I almost wished myself back in the everyday vet's world of dogs and ponies.

Two minutes passed, then five. Suddenly, as if chilled by a gust of icy air, Mary began to tremble. Her knees buckled and she sagged down on legs of jelly. With a drowsy sigh and a boom as her leathery side hit the thick carpet of straw on the floor, she crashed over, flat out, with the operation site and the bad tooth fortuitously uppermost. Matt and Ray Legge, the zoo director, positioned her legs and trunk as comfortably as they could, and I checked her breathing and the working of the massive heart with my stethoscope. The operation was under way.

The peeling back of a large flap of gum over the root area took only a few minutes, and the bleeding was very quickly controlled with forceps. Then began the slow business of chipping away the bone. It was fantastically hard. I struck the sharp chisels with a heavy metal mallet, working to a guideline painted on the bone in purple antiseptic dye. I was working naked from the waist up, as I prefer to do during prolonged large-animal operations, particularly in warm animal houses. The effort was making my arms ache and the sweat streamed down my face and chest. Hordes of little red mites from the straw took it into their heads to climb aboard and stroll about my body, making me itch annoyingly. Bit by bit, but far more slowly than anticipated, I chipped my pathway along the jawbone. It was so hard that the jarring as the mallet and chisel rebounded from the dense tissue began to numb my hands. Mary remained perfectly unconscious. From time to time I stopped my chiselling to examine her pulse and breathing—so far all was well.

After two hours I had at last broken through the jawbone right along the line I had marked. Then, using a strong stainless-steel bone "pin" rather like a small crowbar, I levered the plate of bone off. There below it was the whole of the troublesome molar's complex root system. Like an iceberg, there was far more of the tooth below the surface than protruded above the gum, and the roots were still hideously intertwined with a lacework of bony bridges. On and on I chipped, gradually freeing the broad, curved root branches. With my crowbar I tested my progress now and again by attempting to lever the great tooth outwards. Still it remained firmly implanted. After four hours I could at last see the inflamed area on the root that was the cause of all our problems. It was not much to look at: just a pinkish-yellow blob about the size of a pea. Another hour passed and then, as I tried levering outwards yet again, there was a loud creaking noise and the largest tooth I have ever extracted heeled over and fell out of the jaw with a thud.

From there on it was plain sailing to replace the plate of bone, fill the gaping hole in the gum (it was as big as a house brick) with a four-pound ball of sterilized dental wax, and stitch up. As I began the last lap, replacing the gum flap, I noticed that the gum was not as bright pink in colour as it had been but was now distinctly tinged with lilac. I hurriedly completed the last knots in the catgut and sat back exhausted on my haunches. The colour change in the gum had diluted some of my elation over finishing the job. Now to attend to the animal's general condition and avert possible post-operative complications.

Mary still lay dreaming on her side. Her reflexes were becoming a bit stronger. First I checked the heart and lungs again. Her heart was thumping strongly but faster now. As I listened to her lungs, with the stethoscope placed on the uppermost part of her chest, all sounded normal.

Then, faintly, from far away, I heard the deep rumble of a new sound, a dull bubbling noise far below the healthy *swoosh* of air in and out of the lung nearer to me. I went round to the other side of the animal and knelt down, pushing my stethoscope hard into the tight space between the underneath side of the chest and the floor. I could not get very far in but the bubbling noise was distinct, rather like a cauldron of jam gently boiling. I knew what was beginning to happen. The immense weight of the animal was interfering severely with the flow of air and blood through the vital tissues, and fluid was collecting in the underneath lung. This is something to be watched for in all animals lying on their sides under anaesthetic, and it can usually be prevented by turning the animal frequently from side to side.

"Let's get her over as quickly as possible," I said. "I don't like the sound of the right lung."

Matt and his assistants hurried to attach ropes to Mary's feet and to push planks as levers beneath the bulging belly. Everyone pushed or pulled. Keepers braced themselves with their feet against walls and their backs wedged beneath Mary's legs. Gradually we raised her until she was lying on her backbone with all four feet in the air. Then we let her down gently on the other side. I gave injections of heart and lung stimulants and drugs against shock and infection. The bubbling noise was now less noticeable in the right lung, but to my horror I detected the first sounds of it in the left one. Mary had been down under anaesthetic for too long. Although she was beginning to rouse, she had a long way to go and I had no way of speeding up the process. The lungs were becoming fatigued. We were in trouble. The elephant was beginning to drown.

Mary's breathing became steadily more laboured and abnormal. She was more restless and moved her legs and trunk erratically. She even tried to raise her head a few inches from the ground. The unpleasant sounds in both lungs increased and, more ominously, some areas of the lung tissue became silent; they had filled completely with liquid and there was no longer any movement of air through them. An oxygen cylinder was set up and the gas was fed by tube under a sheet placed over Mary's head. I opened the cylinder valve to the "full on" position. After a few minutes it became painfully clear that, despite the roaring jet of life-giving oxygen blasting into the throat, Mary's breathing was steadily weakening. If only I could reverse the effects of the injected anaesthetic! A full return to consciousness and with it the ability to stand and move would soon have restored good circulation in the chest.

Mary's colour began changing for the worse. The gums were now grey-blue with only a hint of pink. The respiration was weaker and seemed more laboured. The interval between breaths became agonizingly longer.

"Stand next to me and we'll try artificial respiration," I said to Matt, who was standing glum and tight-lipped. "Both together we'll get on and off the chest to see if our weight can compress the ribs."

Simultaneously we both jumped onto the rounded grey chest of the recumbent giant. The rib-cage sank a little. We immediately jumped off again. There was a slight expansion of the chest, but it was impossible to tell how much air had been sucked in. We repeated the process. On, off, on, off—at five-second intervals we jumped with all our weight onto Mary's chest. We tried jumping up and down on the chest itself. Our exertions produced some wheezing as small amounts of air were forced in and out, but it was not enough. I stopped and listened again with the stethoscope. The lungs were in dire trouble, with fluid building up, and the heart was beginning to fail fast. I gave more injections, more circulation stimulant, and a chemical to give a kick in the pants to the centre in the brain that controls breathing. It was no good. Five minutes later Mary stopped breathing altogether and the heartbeats faded away, becoming fainter and fainter until I could hear them no longer. Mary, the most famous of Belle Vue Zoo's elephants and voted by schoolchildren their favourite animal in the park, was dead.

The autopsy on Mary confirmed that the long operation under phencyclidine had produced serious fluid build-up in the lungs with a resulting fatal lack of oxygen and heart failure. The zoo director and I had a meeting with the Board to report on Mary's loss. It was miserable explaining how my technique, up to date as it was, just had not been safe enough for a long operation on an elephant. I told the Board that if another elephant developed the same problem as Mary on the following day I would have to do the same again, using the same drugs. It would be so until someone developed a new way of tackling anaesthesia in the elephant.

It took four long years for that new way to be developed, but fortunately it did materialize, and it came in time to be of use in my next major elephant operation.

I was in Cyprus on holiday with Shelagh and the girls when we saw a large photograph on a Cypriot magazine cover displayed in a bookshop in Nicosia. It showed Billy Smart, Jr., the owner of a troupe of animals whose show performed annually at Flamingo Park, standing in a car-wash with an elephant which was being shampooed in this rather novel way. Prominently visible on the thigh of the animal was a lump the size of a cricket ball. An abscess or a tumour, I remarked to Shelagh. We had no way of knowing when the photograph had been taken; perhaps it was something which had been dealt with long ago. I soon forgot about it.

Two months later the telephone rang. It was Billy Smart, Jr. Gilda, one of his elephant troupe, was having trouble with a strange lump on her hind leg. Apparently the lump, the size of a large apple, had been there for about

a year, but over the past three weeks it had begun to grow
very rapidly and was now as big as a melon. I drove down
to Leicester, where Smart's Circus was playing, and went
into the elephant lines. Sure enough, Gilda was the elephant I had seen in the photograph in Cyprus. The swelling on her leg was hard but apparently painless. Its base
was deep below the skin in the great thigh muscles.

"What do you think it is?" asked Billy. He had had
years of experience with elephants and with the abscesses,
cysts, and skin diseases which are commonly seen in the
species, but he had never seen a lump behaving like this one.

"It doesn't look like an abscess or cyst to me," I replied, exploring the consistency and shape of the thing
with my fingers. "I think it's a tumour."

Billy had trained the elephants himself, and thanks to
his remarkable rapport with them I was able to push a
special biopsy needle deep into the lump in order to sample
the tissue without the animal's reacting or making a fuss:
Billy just stood at Gilda's head, talking firmly and kindly
to her and stroking her trunk while she gazed devotedly
down at him. The speck of flesh on the end of the biopsy
needle was sent to the laboratory for microscopic examination. A few days later the result came back that it was
indeed a tumour, with areas of cancerous change. A major operation to remove it was imperative.

This time the anaesthetic would be a new drug called
M99. I had first used it a few months before on fourteen
young elephants who came to Flamingo Park straight
from the African bush. They were a wild and riotous
bunch and had to be examined carefully; some had weak
and bent ankle joints, and I suspected others of being rup-
tured at the navel. But as soon as I approached closely to
inspect them, they flared their ear flaps and charged at me,
squealing angrily. One young male took such a dislike to

my attentions that he chased me across the elephant house and beat me against the concrete wall with a blow of his broad bony forehead. I literally saw stars. It was obviously going to be necessary to use anaesthetic on these young tearaways if I was to have any chance of giving them a thorough check-up.

I had read good reports about M99 published by vets working with wildlife in Africa and decided to use it on the elephants, even though at that time it cost about £480,000 a pound. It is a powerful drug of the morphine family, and I was assured that only a minute amount—a few milligrammes—would be required for each animal. The most important attribute of the drug was that it could be instantly neutralized by an antidote. I injected each young elephant by a flying dart fired from a special gas-powered rifle. One to two minutes after the dart had struck an elephant's plump buttocks, it sank quietly to the ground without any sign of alarm or dizziness. The medical inspection over, I slipped a small dose of antidote into the ear vein and within two minutes the animal was on its feet, eating food and glaring suspiciously at me once more.

My experiences with M99 and the African elephants had impressed me, but nonetheless I travelled down to Leicester and Gilda again with a slight feeling of apprehension. Everything had been beautifully arranged in the elephant tent for the operation. Deep straw had been piled on the ground and covered with new canvas sheeting. The other elephants had been moved far away to the other end of the tent, where they stood about with a suspicious and disapproving air, watching to see what we were preparing to do to their companion.

Elephants look after one another. They have special friends and mates among their companions from whom, in sickness or health, they are usually inseparable. When I move between two elephants to prod or feel at something they often press together, making me a filling inside an elephant sandwich. It can be difficult to squeeze out, and I usually find myself dropping down and wriggling out between the forest of massive legs. If I inject one elephant, its protective neighbour will often reach out and clout me sternly with its trunk or, worse, if it has tusks, lunge out with the ivory points at my body. One must keep talking gently but firmly, move steadily and decisively, and re-member to bear gifts: Polo mints are very well received.

Gilda had not been given any solid food for twelve hours prior to the operation and was grumbling a bit about this as she was led onto the canvas. She tried to grab bits of straw from the bedding as an illicit snack and became irritable when Billy Smart stopped her.

"I think I'll bring Burma over to stand by her," said Billy. "It will give her more confidence."

Burma is the gorgeous old matriarch of the Smart's Circus elephants. Very big, looking always uniquely old and wise, she is the most intelligent, gentle, and patient elephant I have ever met, just the sort of companion you would want next to you in time of trouble. All the Smarts worship her and see that at Christmas, weddings, and other festivals, or if she looks a little peaky, she receives a bottle or two of her favourite tipple, neat Bisquit de Bouche cognac. The presence of Burma near a nervous, dis-traught, or ailing elephant always seems to bring calm and confidence to the sufferer. I have often been glad of her help when treating sick or injured animals in the Smarts' winter quarters at Winkfield.

Burma came and stood impassively and quietly next to Gilda, who seemed immediately reassured. It was not nec-essary even to drop the anaesthetized elephant onto the floor. Billy simply gave Gilda the command to lie down (this is just one of the advantages of working with circus as opposed to zoo elephants), and the elephant obediently lay down with the tumorous leg uppermost. I could almost hear Burma murmur in approval. It was easy to inject just two cc's of the M99 solution painlessly into Gilda's ear vein, and within half a minute and without any problems she passed from conscious rest into a deep and satisfactory sleep.

It took me about an hour and a half to cut out the great growth. Although elephant skin is tough, it is nothing like as thick and awkward to work with as, say, rhinoceros skin, and ordinary scalpels cut through it with the greatest of ease. The time-consuming part was the tying off of all the blood vessels that supplied the hidden depths of the tumour.

When at last the mass had been totally dissected out (I had been at great pains not to leave behind even one particle that might multiply into another tumour), there was left a gaping hole in the thigh which had to be closed. It was virtually impossible to slide the skin across the hole, because the gap was so large and I had been forced to remove a great expanse of skin. For a moment I was frightened. The hole had to be closed, but how? Using double lengths of the thickest stitch material I had, a sort of plaited nylon fishing line with a breaking strain of 250 pounds, I inserted "relaxation sutures," which go through the skin far behind the wound edges and take the main strain. I put dozens of them in place and gradually tightened them. Slowly the wound began to close. As the first relaxation sutures went slack I tightened them and reinforced with more.

At last it was finished. The hole was sealed, although the operation site looked like a spider's web of interweaving green nylon. I prayed it would be strong enough to withstand the pressures when Gilda moved about. After tidying up the wound I filled my syringe with the anaesthetic antidote, injected it into the ear vein, and looked at my watch. Thirty seconds later Gilda sighed deeply, switched her trunk, and rolled her eyes. Then she heaved herself over onto her brisket and with a little grunt rose to her feet. No wobbling, no dizziness. Gilda looked round, touched trunks briefly with Burma, and then grabbed a tuft of straw protruding from beneath the canvas and stuffed it hungrily into her mouth. The stitches held.

There was no further trouble with Gilda and her tumour. The last sign of it was the faint white scar which could just be detected the following Christmas when I sat with Shelagh and watched Smart's Circus on television. The audience in the big top and the millions of television viewers undoubtedly enjoyed the scintillating display as the elephants carried clowns and glamorous girls about the ring. But the glimpse of that thin and fading line on the prancing grey hams of an elephant made me the proudest person on earth that Boxing-day afternoon.

11 Foreign Bodies

IN SPITE OF THE FACT that continual progress is being made in animal anaesthesia, with new drugs and improved methods of delivering them being developed every year, the giraffe is still one of the most difficult animals to knock out successfully. The whole process is fraught with danger: Evolution's gift of a long neck has also burdened the species with a peculiar tendency for its blood pressure to go out of control under general anaesthesia, and that fragile neck, with its specialized anatomy, is also liable to injury once the animal is rendered unconscious.

One day soon after Andrew had joined the practice I received another call from Windsor Safari Park, outside London: A big male giraffe had begun to limp. I drove down from Rochdale to have a look at him and saw immediately that the trouble was in one forefoot; there was a puffy, angry-looking swelling bulging out above the hoof. I decided to have a feel at it.

Tempting the giraffe with apples, we led him into the special "giraffe crush" we had had built so that I could take blood samples, do minor operations under local anaesthetic, give injections, and, as is frequently necessary, trim overgrown toenails with an electric saw, chisels, and a sanding machine. The animals were so accustomed to being held in the device, which didn't hurt or upset them, that I had even found it possible to take blood pressure readings by inserting a needle into the carotid artery. Because of the relaxed demeanour and calm state of the animals, my results were probably the first accurate measurements of their kind ever made on normal, unstressed, untranquillized giraffes. (In fact, these measurements had revealed that giraffes run a normally high blood pressure.)

On this occasion when I gently touched the swollen foot the pain must have been intense, for the bull giraffe reacted violently and kicked back mightily with a hind leg. The leg struck the heavy metal framework which formed the gate into the "crush," knocking the whole two tons of metal from its hinges as if it were made of paper. As the steel gate broke away I jumped back from where I was crouching, missed my footing, and stumbled as the great framework toppled towards me. With great presence of mind, Gary Smart, one of the directors of the park who was standing nearby, flung himself at me, literally cannoning me out from under, and the gate crashed with a metallic roar onto the concrete floor inches from my body. But for Gary it would have crippled or killed me.

Having dusted myself off, I continued my examination. Something had badly infected the foot, but I could find no puncture wound or any sign of an irritant piece of flint or cinder trapped in the sensitive flesh between the animal's two toes. I decided to treat the inflammatory condition with injections of antibiotics and to combine this with soothing poultices of magnesium sulphate paste. Every day the injections were repeated and the poultices faithfully applied. The redness went out of the foot swelling, but it stayed enlarged, and the giraffe continued to limp pitifully. Pain-killers didn't help, nor did having a keeper stand all day hosing the affected digits with hot water.

A week passed, and then two, and I saw that the swelling was concentrating in one of the two toes. Still the giraffe hobbled painfully. I was getting desperate. I resorted to intravenous sulpha drugs and then to those antibiotics which had special powers of penetrating bone, and others which could deal with bugs that had developed resistance to penicillin or tetracyclines. It was beginning to look as though the bone of the toe was diseased, a condition for which there is no hope of a purely medical cure.

For the first time I began to consider surgery. It was a daunting prospect—amputating the toe, a sizable object weighing ten pounds or more, of an animal renowned as being disastrously difficult to anaesthetize successfully—and a very tough decision. The animal was valuable and had been siring some superb youngsters. Suppose my diagnosis was incorrect? Suppose I took the toe off and dissected it only to find healthy bone with the infection limited to the soft tissues? And what about the technical problems apart from the anaesthesia: the difficulty of daily dressings, the sheer size of the operation site? How long could I afford to keep the giraffe down and out? How would a giraffe fare, getting about on just one toe?

One of the great benefits of working as a zoo vet is that the owners with which one has to deal are themselves professionals. They have economic objectives but they are humane and genuinely care for their stock. They rarely exhibit the misguided sentimentality or the hysteria sometimes seen in owners of domestic dogs and cats when sickness or accident strikes their pets. I outlined the position to the directors at Windsor and explained how I had arrived at my opinion that the giraffe's foot was concealing a focus of intractable diseased tissue deep within the bone itself. I also explained the uncertainties and the dangers of the operation. I got an unqualified go-ahead. Windsor and I had fought to save sick or injured animals ranging from lizards right up to their prized killer whale. We had lost some bouts but won a good many others, and I think they trusted me. That is something of which I am still rather proud, for the people who own Windsor Safari Park have years of top-class animal experience behind them as owners of the internationally famous Billy Smart's Circus.

I was not going to run at the thing bald-headed. I planned the whole operation for several days and decided that I would have to have Andrew with me to share the burden. His knowledge of physiology is unsurpassed. With him at the head end to look after the anaesthetized giraffe, monitoring the vital processes and if necessary intervening here or there with supportive drugs and electrical instruments, I could concentrate on the purely surgical matter of cutting off the diseased half of the foot as quickly as possible. It was going to be quite an affair. I would need lots of keepers, dozens of bales of straw, and a formidable collection of equipment.

A few days before the operation I had a look at the foot and found that a ragged gap had appeared between the top of the hoof and the flesh of the toe. Nothing much was coming out, but it reassured me that we had indeed a case of deep bone infection on our hands.

On the day of the operation Andrew arrived from the north with his usual complement of white-coated disciples, all of them excited at the prospect of having an off-beat case to add to their clinical notebooks. They set up an electrocardiograph with which Andrew would keep track of the heart function during the operation. The giraffe stood in a special pen with padded sides and a floor deeply covered in straw, calmly chewing his cud and superciliously watching us scurry about below.

Eventually I was ready. Everything was in place: instruments, dressings, buckets of water, drugs, oxygen, emergency equipment, ropes, and a full complement of reliable keepers. I began by giving the giraffe a tranquillizing injection, then followed with a small but potent dose of Immobilon, a special combination of M99 together with a long-acting sedative.

We all stood silently looking up at the bull. I thought about the globule of yellow liquid swirling steadily up the ten feet to those long-lashed eyes, now gazing patronizingly down at us. I imagined the first molecules of Immobilon streaming down the blood vessels of the brain, clambering out through the walls like so many office workers leaving a tube train at rush hour, and paralysing the brain cells. Seconds later the stately animal rocked once on his feet and then collapsed with the suddenness and silence of a tent whose guy ropes are cut.

As soon as the giraffe was flat out on the ground, Andrew dashed in and attached his electrodes for the electrocardiograph. His little band of disciples swarmed like white bats around the front end and half a dozen stethoscopes began maintaining a listening watch. I decided to forget about the animal and the anaesthesia. They would be in good hands with my partner. For me there was only The Foot.

Having checked to be sure that the animal was completely insensible to pain, I scrubbed, shaved, and disinfected the whole of the troublesome leg with the aid of a couple of keepers. For the amputation I was going to use a flexible wire saw, an elegant and simple method which has the great advantage of speed. The saw consists of a length of wire with a stainless-steel handle attached at each end. Pulled back and forth between the two hands in a strong, steady, rapid movement, the instrument will cut through the densest of materials. As it moves the wire generates much friction and heat, which automatically cauterizes and seals all but the largest blood vessels in its path. There are problems, however. For one thing it is a procedure requiring a great deal of effort, particularly when cutting through a bone as thick as the one in a giraffe's foot. If my arms were to tire during the sawing, the reduced friction and consequent lowering of heat production might allow a haemorrhage. The wire saw also requires considerable skill to guide it along a prearranged route with several changes of direction.

I decided to check any haemorrhage that might result from my tiring by fixing a kind of tourniquet. I tied a thick strip of automobile inner-tube rubber round the upper part of the leg and tested the arterial pulse. It was barely perceptible below the tourniquet. Now I must finish the job within half an hour to avoid damage to the leg by oxygen lack.

I put my wire saw in place between the two toes, grasped the stainless-steel handles, and began sawing, as keepers held the leg steady. I had already taken the precaution of stripping down to a pair of swimming trunks; I knew this was going to be an immensely sweaty affair. Left-right, left-right, left-right. The wire cut through the soft tissues like butter. On I went, cleaving an easy path between the toes, until I met the first sign of resistance. I was hitting bone. Perspiring freely, I increased the power and speed of my sawing and was pleased to see puffs of smoke coming up from the operation site. There was no sign of blood; I was cutting and sealing the bone.

I laboured on until eventually I had gone above the area of inflammation. Now came the tricky part. Without slackening the pace I had to angle outwards, cutting right across the thick dense part of the outer half of the foot and making for the skin. The keepers strained to hold the leg firmly as I and my wire pulled violently against them.

My arms and my back began to ache violently. Sweat poured down my forehead and swept like stinging rain into my eyes. I became dizzy with the left-to-right swing of my body. Of one thing only was I aware: I must not stop or slacken for an instant or the smoke and the smell of frying bone might be replaced by a welter of blood.

I kept the rhythm up and in an agonized contortion bent down to look at the undersurface of the leg. My sawing position seemed to be OK. The line of the cut was well above the diseased zone. Left-right, left-right. Would I ever get through the bone? Then with a thrill I saw that the expanse of skin between the two ends of the smoking wire was rapidly getting smaller. I would soon be through the toe and have only a little bit of skin to sever! I made one exhausted and desperate burst of speed. The wire zinged through the final millimetre of bone, shot through the skin, and broke away. I crashed backwards head over heels into the straw. Done!

I sat up and looked at the great naked area of tissue which I had exposed, scanning it anxiously for any signs of infection or inflammation. If I had not cut completely through clean tissue the condition might well travel right up the leg. But I could see no sign of trouble.

"The heart's beginning to flutter a bit," Andrew said. "How long will you be?" He was preparing to shoot something into the animal's jugular vein.

"Can you give just ten minutes more?" I asked. "That should be long enough for me to put on a good dressing."

Before doing anything I released the pressure of the tourniquet for a second to see what the effect would be. A little blood began to ooze from the cut surface where the toe had been removed; it was not enough to warrant spending time to search for and ligature tiny arteries. I would go ahead with the simple pressure dressing.

I sprayed the raw tissue with antibiotics and covered it

thickly with Vaseline-coated gauze, then applied thick
wedges of cotton wool and strapped them down by tight
bandaging. Removing the tourniquet altogether, I waited
for a minute to see whether or not the renewed flow of
blood would pump its way through. The bandages stayed
white so I pressed on. I had chosen plaster of Paris to form
the final outer coat of the dressing. As fast as I could, I
wound reel after reel of the soaked plaster bandages around
the whole of the foot while a keeper blew hot air onto
them from a hair dryer to speed up setting. Finally it was
done, and it only remained for me to waterproof the whole
thing by painting it briskly with a special lacquer.

"We must finish now," said Andrew. He was looking
anxiously at the paper trace that flowed continually from
the electrocardiograph. "He's not responding any more
to the Pastrum." This is a German circulatory stimulant
that has saved the day for me at countless operations.

"It's OK," I said. "Go ahead and give the reviver.
Get him up as quick as you like!"

The instrument trolleys and electrocardiograph were
wheeled out of the way.

"Everybody out now!" I shouted. It would take only
a few seconds for the anaesthetic antidote to work, and I
didn't want anybody getting trodden on.

While I watched, Andrew injected a small quantity
of blue liquid into the jugular vein. We waited. Thirty
seconds later the giraffe gave a pleasant sigh as if a delightful dream had just ended and began to breathe much more
deeply. Andrew listened to the chest with his stethoscope,
smiled, and gave me a thumbs-up signal. Another minute
passed and then suddenly as if some fairy godmother had
waved her wand the sleeping fellow opened his eyes,
raised his long neck, looked backwards over his body,
flicked his ears, and then gracefully slipped up into a stand-

ing position. Without a trace of grogginess he looked round for something to eat. It was marvellous to see him curl his long grey tongue round a banana and chomp it up with relish. Most pleasing of all was the obvious fact that for the first time in weeks he was putting all his weight on the foot where the toe had been removed. The pain had gone at last!

Later in the day after a shower and a few beers, Andrew and I took the amputated toe up to the laboratory and sawed it in half. Right in the middle of the bone we found a small piece of steel surrounded by pus and dead tissue. Somehow this foreign body had burrowed through the skin or possibly the hoof wall, which had closed behind it, leaving no trace. It had worked its way into the bone, where it had set up the unyielding processes of infection and inflammation. Before we travelled north later that evening we pickled the halves of the amputated toe and presented them to the Safari Park's museum. Two weeks after the operation I doped the giraffe again and cut off the dressing. Everything had healed perfectly, and I felt great when I saw the now-seven-toed bull giraffe walk off proudly and without a trace of a limp into the sunlight.

That bit of steel got into the giraffe's foot when he trod on it, but more often foreign objects are introduced into zoo animals by their swallowing them. The elephant at Belle Vue Zoo that took an umbrella did not seem to suffer the slightest twinge of the collywobbles, although an enormous old elephant seal at Cleethorpes found a woolly cardigan too much for it and tragically choked to death. Sometimes, of course, these things are ingested accidentally, but at other times there may be special reasons for them being taken in voluntarily.

The sea-lion, for example, can often be found in the wild carrying a few stones quite harmlessly in its stomach. These stones act as ballast to help the animal dive, rather like the weighted belt of a skin diver; thus, deeper-diving species of sea-lion tend to carry more ballast than shallower-diving ones. In captivity this natural, fairly limited taking on of stones can go wrong. Where sea-lions are kept in fresh water with no access to salt, particularly if the pool is a simple one scooped out of the earth, the animal may attempt to satisfy its craving for salt in its diet by eating soil and stones. To avoid this I try to see that all the sea-lions and seals in my care that are not in saltwater pools have table salt added daily to their fish diet.

Unfortunately, I still see the results of stone-swallowing by sea-lions over a long period, as when a sea-lion at a safari park in England died suddenly after a lengthy spell of erratic eating. For months it had been keen to feed but quickly lost its appetite after being given one or two fish; then it would be hungry again within half an hour. The owners had not worried unduly because the sea-lion seemed to be gaining weight. Indeed it was!

When I looked at the body it had a plump rounded belly that should surely be full of fat. I began the autopsy and within seconds of slicing through the abdominal wall was faced with an amazing sight. The stomach, which is normally about the same size and shape as a human's and lies tucked neatly away under the rib-cage, was horribly distended. It filled the abdomen, squeezing the liver and kidneys and intestines. It bulged everywhere, particularly back towards the tail. I could not see the end of it; it continued on into the pelvic cavity, where only the bladder and associated organs should be found. Inside the stomach were stones, hundreds and hundreds of them, packing every bit of available space and stretching the stomach wall

until it was as thin as tissue paper. When they were all
removed they filled three gallon buckets and weighed almost forty pounds. It was the worst foreign-body load I
had ever seen.

There were other sea-lions in the safari park of the
same age as the poor dead individual. What about them?
They were fit-looking animals that delighted in performing their skilful feats of balance before the visitors. All
looked well, but I was of a mind to X-ray the lot of them
to make certain that no more were carrying around stom-
achs like gravel pits. I asked the trainer whether there
were any other abnormal symptoms to report.

He thought for a moment and began to shake his
head. "No, I don't think so, except . . ."–he frowned and
then went on–"except for Mimi. She's a little bit like
Otto, the dead one, always hungry but very easily filled."

I walked over to where Mimi stood elegantly on her
show stand. She sniffed diffidently at me and clapped her
front flippers hopefully. I could see no sign of trouble
brewing. Then the trainer called Mimi off the stand and
she slipped down onto the ground and hauled herself
towards the fish bucket. As she passed I heard a soft and
unusual sound like the lapping of water on a shingle beach,
the rush of pebbles one upon another. There was too
much incidental noise from the other animals and the visitors to hear it clearly, so I had Mimi taken to the quiet of
the hospital. There I listened again. When she moved it
was possible to hear the crunching, grinding noise of
gravel. I stroked her and made friends and then carefully
pressed her stomach. *Scr-r-runch*. It was exactly like
digging into a bag of marbles. Mimi was full of rocks.

Along with the giraffe, the sea-lion is one of the more
difficult animals to anaesthetize. It responds unpredictably
to the whole range of injectable anaesthetics, and its

ability to hold its breath makes the use of anaesthetic gases problematic. Nonetheless, I decided to operate. I would use heavy doses of the safest sea-lion tranquillizer I knew plus extensive local injections of novocaine. Opening the stomach of a dog to remove swallowed objects is a common and not very difficult operation, but the sea-lion is somewhat trickier. A particular risk is post-operative infection from the skin, which literally teems with all sorts of nasty bacteria. For the surgeon, too, contact with sea-lion skin and other tissues can be risky if there are any cuts in his rubber gloves and abrasions on his hands. A germ often found living harmlessly on sea-lion skin can attack pigs, dolphins, and other animals dramatically and in humans may set up the unpleasant infection known to generations of seal skinners and whaling men as "blubber finger" or "seal hand."

From Mimi's stomach I retrieved 124 stones weighing almost sixteen pounds altogether. No wonder she had been hungry, with nowhere to accommodate a decent meal! When she was stitched up, Mimi was a much more streamlined creature. I looked forward to seeing her eat a hearty meal of three or four pounds of herring in a few days after the stomach sutures had done their work and she could come off the post-operative diet of liquefied fish and water.

It is not always necessary to approach the stomach by cutting through the abdomen. Increasingly nowadays, particularly in dolphins, arch-swallowers of bric-à-brac, we employ an ingenious piece of equipment normally used for exploring the higher reaches of the human bowel, the Olympus fibre-optic gastroscope.

This is a very expensive device which can do wonders when slipped simply and without anaesthetic down the animal's throat. It is thin and flexible and carries a powerful light source, a mobile viewing tip, a water spray, an air tube for inflating organs to be inspected, and a host of special attachments. Looking through the eyepiece we can see magnified and in full colour every nook and cranny in the stomach and even farther down into the intestine or up the bile duct. The tip can be made to go round corners and to look backwards towards the viewer. By passing minute instruments down within the tube we can cauterize bleeding points, take biopsy samples of diseased tissue, and grab or lasso objects. The stomach and bowels expanded by air from the gastroscope become fascinating caverns and grottoes through which by remote control we can wander in search of the bizarre and the diseased.

One of the first patients on which we used the fibre-optic gastroscope was Brandy, a talented star of the dolphin show at Marineland in Palma Nova, Majorca. One day, for no apparent reason, Brandy swallowed one of the soft plastic rings, six inches across, which he played with during his performances. Down into his stomach it went, and down it stayed. Nothing untoward happened at first, and Brandy continued to eat and work normally. But the powerful acids in his stomach slowly vulcanized the plastic and began to turn the soft ring into something much more hard and irritant. David Mudge, the director of Marineland and an old friend in the dolphin business, became worried when the ring was not regurgitated as he had hoped. What was more, after some days Brandy began to look unwell. He was irritable, his work became erratic, and his appetite disappeared. David was certain that Brandy was experiencing stomach pain.

We had talked together over the telephone when the ring was first swallowed and had decided to observe the animal and to treat him conservatively at first. Now it became obvious that we would have to intervene with strong

positive measures. Andrew flew out to Majorca with the
fibre-optic gastroscope, accompanied by David Wild, the
most skilled "driver," as he calls himself, of the complex
instrument in the country. Brandy certainly looked ill. He
was pale, seemed tense and in pain, and his usual cheeky,
vivacious temperament had changed to one of irritable
misery. No longer was he cock of the male dolphins in
Palma Nova, forever paying court to his harem of admiring females. Blood analysis showed strong evidence of
bleeding ulcers in his stomach. Without further ado Brandy
was caught, hauled out of the pool, and placed on a soft
rubber mattress.

Like whales, dolphins out of water produce a lot of
body heat and, unless they are kept wet, may overheat and
show dangerous cracking and peeling of the skin. A man
stood by with a bucket, wetting the animal down while
Andrew completed his preparations. First, wet towels were
wrapped round Brandy's upper and lower jaws and used
to pull the mouth open and hold it open. Gently, Andrew
passed the lubricated gastroscope over the back of the dolphin's tongue, to one side of the larynx, and then down
the gullet into the first stomach. Kneeling behind him
David Wild watched through the eyepiece as the tip of the
instrument moved onwards, spraying the lens with water
when stomach juices threatened to cloud the vision and
pushing the walls of the stomach away from the tube with
air so that he could have space to look around. Through a
side attachment to the eyepiece Andrew was able to
monitor progress as well.

Before long they both saw the first of a series of ugly
bleeding ulcers in the stomach lining. Everywhere there
was black blood from the ulcers, partly digested. Brandy's
stomach was in a terrible state. David swung the tip of the
gastroscope round, so they could see a segment of red plas-

tic lying in a black pool of blood. There was the ring! The natural contractions of the stomach muscles against the hardening ring were grinding one ulcer after another through the delicate velvety lining of the organ.

Now to get the ring out. A special attachment to the gastroscope allowed the introduction of a wire loop which was guided round the ring and back to the gastroscope again. When the ring was firmly snared it was pulled to the tip of the instrument, and then both ring and gastroscope were withdrawn together. Brandy gave an enormous gulp as the ring travelled back up. Luckily, dolphins have remarkably elastic gullets for swallowing large fish whole, or there would have been the risk of a rupture.

With the ring gone Brandy looked much relieved, but Andrew reintroduced the gastroscope to inspect the ulcer damage. Some of the worst bleeding points were electrically cauterized and photographs were taken. Then Brandy was returned, to his great relief, to the pool and his wives, his complete recovery ensured by a course of tablets normally given to dyspeptic middle-aged business executives. To celebrate his sense of well-being after the poolside operation, Brandy was seen to mate long and amorously with one of the female dolphins, and eleven and a half months later, on the following Boxing-day, a little baby dolphin was born in the pool at Palma Nova.

12 The Amazing Performing Dolphin Doctor

As I have observed earlier, one of the rewards of being a zoo vet is the caliber of many of the people one meets in the course of one's work. The owners, zoo directors, keepers, and trainers who are responsible for the animals I treat have often developed a deep rapport with their charges; after years of living and working together their knowledge of the animals is instinctual.

Typical of these skilled and humane animal trainers are the members of the Naumann family from Germany. They travel all over the world with their big cats, and I have spent many hours watching them train their lions, tigers, and pumas. They raise their cats from cubs and work patiently long hours each day, teaching the animals to perform by reward—in the form of finger-sized pieces of tender meat or in stroking, patting, and praise.

By these methods the Naumanns created a unique high-diving tiger act, in which a fully grown Bengal tiger dived into a circular swimming pool from a platform twenty feet above the water. Several years ago the Naumanns arrived in Manchester with all their gear and their cats for a summer season in the grounds at Belle Vue. Work went ahead to assemble the pool, ladder, and platform.

Everything was set up—but not exactly to order. Somehow the platform was not positioned directly over the centre of the pool as it should have been. This mistake was not apparent to anyone looking from below. Nor, it seems, did the tiger realize anything was wrong when he climbed up the ladder for his first Manchester performance and, after suitable fanfares and drum rolls, launched himself into the air.

The flying tiger plunged down into the water but in landing rapped his back sharply against the metal edge of the pool. In great pain and partially paralysed, the poor animal struggled out of the water and dragged himself to his trainer. The Naumanns were understandably distraught at the pain caused to one of their beloved cats by the carelessness of a member of their team. Within minutes I arrived at the scene to examine the patient, and Shelagh came with me, as she occasionally does if she's not busy.

The accident had produced bleeding and severe tissue damage in the canal carrying the spinal cord down the lower back. The pressure of the blood and swollen soft tissues was pinching the nerve within its bony passageway, and as every minute passed the tiger was suffering more pain in the spine and losing the use of his hind legs. The front end of the animal was distinctly aggrieved and in a foul temper. Whatever might be the case with the two hind feet, the front two and the jaws were in fine fettle. We would have to handle the tiger in his small travelling cage, to which he had been gently carried immediately after the accident. This was where the kindness and patience of Herr Naumann in training his animals personally from the time they were tiny cubs paid off.

"Don't worry," he said to me, opening the little door into the cage. "You will be able to do whatever you need. I will look after that."

He squeezed through the opening into the cage and beckoned me to follow. I went in and Herr Naumann's wife closed the door and locked it behind us. Shelagh was standing outside with a trace of apprehension on her face. There was not much room inside. The tiger lay growling and groaning in pain, his tail lying limply, too numb to be switched.

Naumann went to the animal and knelt down. Affectionately he took the tiger's head in his hands and brought it onto his lap. He stroked it and talked soothingly in German. The tiger stopped growling and lay impassively.

"Go ahead," said the trainer. "He'll be OK now."

Inwardly I marvelled at his confidence. If there were any fractures waiting for my probing fingers, disturbance of the tortured tissues might well make the animal feel anything but OK. Very gingerly I placed my hands on the muscular back of the big cat, pressing gradually deeper into the tissues, feeling for the spine, tracing the outlines of the vertebrae, and running down the sides of the pelvis. The tiger tensed whenever I came across damaged areas and sometimes growled. At his head, Naumann tightened his embrace.

The next stage was more delicate. I wanted to feel the inside contours of the pelvis as far as possible, which meant putting two fingers deep inside the anus. I slipped on a finger stall, lubricated my hand, and slowly introduced my fingers into the rectum—the first and I suppose the only time that I will ever do that to a conscious adult tiger. The tiger growled and wriggled his front end a bit. He was not amused by this approach, but I was able to satisfy myself that there were no palpable pelvic fractures. It looked as if the lower spine had only been badly bruised and jarred. With any luck the soft tissue swelling could be dispelled and the spinal cord would in time return to its normal function.

I prepared injections of pain-killers, inflammation shrinkers, and enzymes to speed the removal of damaged cells and blood clots. Naumann continued to murmur reassuringly to the tiger while I selected new sharp disposable needles. If there was going to be a sudden nasty reaction it would surely be now. I glanced at Naumann's face, only an inch away from the cat's curved fangs. One short-distance blow from the left forefoot would open up his chest like a fork impaling boiled ham. Gritting my teeth, I indicated to Naumann that I was about to strike.

"Go ahead," he said again. "He understands we're not here to tease him."

I stabbed the needle as quickly as I could through the tough skin and deep into the muscle. To my relief the tiger was apparently unaware of the injection and did not stir. Eventually all the drugs were safely inside him. We left the cage and discussed the setting up of an infra-red lamp above the patient's back and the preparation of my favourite invalid food for sick big cats, a sort of steak tartare made of minced steak, raw egg, dried milk powder, and sterilized bone flour.

The next day the tiger was more comfortable but still largely paralysed at the rear, which was causing secondary constipation. It would be necessary to give him an enema. I made up a small pail of warm water and soap flakes and primed an ordinary human enema pump. Once again Naumann cradled the head of the tiger in his arms while I filled the rear up with the soapy solution. Soon I was gratified to be covered in an explosive eruption of froth and tiger excrement, to the apparent relief of the tiger.

Each day the tiger made more and more progress towards recovery. Little by little the power of his hind legs returned, although the sluggish bowel action remained for almost two weeks.

As the animal became more mobile we had more diffi-

culty in giving the enema. He would rise to his feet with me
and my pump still attached to his rectum and, leaving Naumann behind, would spin round in the small cage in an effort to reach the person doing embarrassing things to his
stern. Until Naumann could catch up with the head again
and return it firmly to his lap, I had to keep myself, pumping wildly away with one hand and dragging my slopping
pail with the other, as close to the animal's bottom as possible. As long as I spun round in the constricted space and
did not let the stern get away from me, the cat could not
quite reach me with tooth or claw. If the cage had been
any larger, constipation might well have triumphed.

At last the enemas were over, and a heap of laxative
breakfast cereal sliced into the patient's meat for a few days
was all that was needed. The tiger made a complete recovery, and when I was satisfied that he was a hundred per-
cent up to scratch I let him go back to the diving board.

Although many circus animals are trained without
cruelty, there are still a few terrible black spots. You will
find them in the smaller, tatty circuses and menageries if you
can penetrate the closed, suspicious, obstructive world behind the scenes. It is a world skilled in repelling outsiders
and deceiving humane society inspectors and, most important, able to move on if trouble is brewing. At first hand I
have seen bears encouraged to move from travelling box to
circus ring by flaming newspapers being thrust underneath
them, and I have heard the regular, sickening thuds as a
chained African elephant was beaten systematically with
bamboo rods by two keepers to break it by literally tor-
turing it until it collapsed. The most repellent feature of
the process was the calm clinical way in which the keepers
administered the beating. It was a job, just like grooming,
which called for a repetitive movement for long periods of

time: no anger, no emotion, just a boring job of beating. Of course, when the police arrived the men were indeed grooming the elephant. Bamboo rods applied with all a man's might across the rib-cage of an elephant leave no marks.

One hard-bitten old lion trainer showed me his method for giving pills to lions. "Watch this, young fella," he said, running the big male lion into the barred tunnel between ring and travelling cage. "Quicker and better than all your dart-guns and powders on the meat."

When the lion was halfway down the tunnel the trainer slipped a board between the bars in front of him and a similar one behind to make a simple treatment cage. He picked up a crowbar and a bottle of aspirins, shoved the crowbar through the bars, and cracked it hard down on the animal's head. The lion was at the trainer's mercy, unable to back away or turn round. He roared thunderously, opening his jaws and raising his head. The lion trainer dropped in a couple of aspirins. Down they went and the lion closed his mouth. The trainer hit the lion's skull again. The sound was sharp and revolting, the clang of metal on bone. The lion roared again in frantic impotence. Two more aspirins went in.

"See? How's that, eh?" said the trainer proudly. "No problem, eh?"

"Bloody horrible," I replied. He would never understand.

At another circus I watched an act purporting to be a chimpanzees' tea party where the animals were not just as good as gold, they were almost automatons. The audience marvelled at the obedience of the little apes and smiled as the trainer fondled their hairy heads. It was all in the fondling. The man showed me his thumbnail, which had been allowed to grow long and then filed into a vicious point. It was strong and horny, and he used it with cruel skill to gouge and twist the sensitive flaps of the chimpanzees' ears. It was really a display of brutal sleight-of-hand carried on in full view of the public. I was to find that this method of controlling chimps by their delicate ears was commonplace in the world of chimpanzee training; even mature specimens were subdued by the agony of a quickly applied hold.

There will always be some showman who is prepared to use inhumane methods to create a new crowd puller. At one marineland in the United States the high spot of the show was a water-skiing elephant. I was there on the day that the elephant was persuaded by a lavish use of the feathered spike to mount a pair of specially constructed giant skis. His rolling, anxious eyes and shrill trumpeting showed clearly that the elephant was an unwilling amphibian—so unwilling that once in position he was chained to the skis and the chains were secured not by padlocks, as is usual when tethering elephants, but by heavy nuts and bolts. To the applause of the crowd and the smooth spiel of the loudspeakers the motorboat towing the skiing elephant pulled away onto the smooth water of the lake. The animal waved his trunk and seemed to hang back on the chains. The skis tipped up at the front as the boat accelerated.

"Look at Herbie go, folks!" enthused the loudspeakers. "My, he's sure enjoying himself!"

The skis were supported beneath by large buoyancy chambers so Herbie did not have to do much in the way of balancing. The boat accelerated into a turn. Herbie's ears flapped in the wind and he waved his trunk more furiously. It must have been too tight a turn. With a mighty crash and an eruption of white water, Herbie lurched over with a squeal of despair and capsized into the lake. Only the upturned bottoms of the ski floats were to be seen. Somewhere under the surface, still chained to the skis, was Herbie. I struggled through the horrified crowds with the vet attached to the marineland, but by the time we had got round to the point on the lakeside closest to the scene of the accident it was too late. Boats had gone out and found Herbie drowned. Without the chains he would have stood a good chance.

Since the principles of good management of performing animals are frequently ignored in the richer, so-called advanced countries, perhaps one should not be surprised that in countries where poverty forces a lower value on human life itself the treatment of exotic animals in captivity would send an appalled shudder through a vet or any other animal lover.

To dolphins the Far East recently has been like Devil's Island to French convicts; once arrived there they rarely return alive. There has been a lucrative business, largely organized by German theatrical agents, sending pairs of European dolphins out on tours of Thailand, the Philippines, Indonesia, Singapore, and Taiwan. Asians adore circuses, travelling shows, and novelty exhibitions, particularly where animals are involved. The "intelligent giant fish," which I believe a majority of the audiences confuse with the feared shark, is immensely popular. The Flipper series of TV shows has been broadcast widely in the Far East and has heightened the interest; every travelling dolphin show naturally has as one of its performers "the original Flipper direct from Florida, U.S.A."

A typical tour is organized in this fashion: A theatrical agent in, say, Munich agrees to provide a team of performing dolphins to a sponsor in Singapore. The deal, which can run into many hundreds of thousands of dollars, is worked out between the German agent's Singapore representative and the sponsor, who is almost invariably an overseas Chinese. The Chinese sponsor then sells pieces of the show to other Chinese in Taiwan or Thailand, who in turn may sell or sublet portions of their shares to still more individuals or syndicates. Now the German agent, with a fat contract in his pocket and an advance payment in the bank and with frequently only a few weeks' time, has to find an owner of performing dolphins who is willing to lease them out.

Because of the cash involved and the tight deadline, the owners of the dolphins are promised the earth if they will send a couple of animals accompanied by a trainer to what, it is emphatically assured, will be a relaxed working holiday in the sunshine. No expense will be spared in fulfilling any of the owners' requirements if only they will come up with the goods and see that the animals present themselves at such and such an airport on a certain day. Transport? No problem. A chartered jet all the way. Water? Nothing to worry about. Everyone knows there's plenty of water in Indonesia and Singapore and the Philippines. Think of those tropical islands set in limpid blue seas! Fish? You could not imagine places richer in the harvest of the sea. Don't people out there subsist largely on fish diets? Think of the millions of little fishing boats that swarm around Hong Kong!

The problems arise when the dolphin trainer and his pair of greased and trussed-up dolphins start out for the Far East. The contracts with their acres of small print don't help much when—after a short and satisfactory first leg of the flight from, say, Paris to Luxembourg on a cargo jet —a transfer is made to an ancient Dakota that will continue the rest of the route. The theatrical agent has been doing some homework and has arrived at the not very surprising conclusion that his profit would be that much plumper if a propeller plane stopping perhaps ten times or more along the way was used instead of a non-stop 707. So the journey might take five days instead of twenty-four hours? Well, they can have a good rest for a couple of days before starting shows when they get to their destination, and the trainer can feed the dolphins on board during the flight, can't he? And if he needs some more water for the fish (I beg your pardon, of course they're dolphins, not fish), he can pick it up easily enough when they're shifting freight at Rome or Athens or Cairo or Karachi or Calcutta or Rangoon or Saigon. Won't it do 'em good to get some sun on their backs on the airfield at Bangkok where they have to be unloaded for three or four hours in order to get off the wooden crates of machinery which had been packed behind them?

So gay little Atlantic bottle-nosed dolphins find themselves in the back yards of Buddhist temples in Singapore's Chinatown, up in the sweating hills of Borneo, or slipped into the bill of a wrestling championship held in a football stadium in downtown Manila. It is bad enough for the human attendants, who arrive haggard and exhausted after half a week in the air. But what must the dolphins be experiencing, out of water, unfed, bumped and jarred, and subjected to rapid changes in temperature, humidity, and air pressure for the same length of time? At journey's end, unlike their trainer, they still wear their fixed and cheeky grin, and the protective grease that envelops them masks any bruises or bedsores. Nor can any damage done to internal organs by the weight of a body deprived of the evenly distributed support of sea water for so many long hours be assessed with the naked eye. It may be days before the serious results are manifestly apparent.

But their troubles are not over by any means once they

arrive in Asia. The pool may be still unfinished, the water as black as ink and in short supply, clean salt unobtainable, the species of fish provided too small or too large and all rotten, and the electricity, if it is on at all, subject to such violent fluctuations in voltage that the fuses in the filter pump blow half a dozen times a day and the water in consequence becomes fouler.

Theoretically, the local representative of the theatrical agent is on hand to iron out all problems and make everyone's stay a happy one, making sure that there is a small refrigerator in working order in the fish kitchen, rooting about for spare fuses for the filter pump, finding good accommodations for the trainer, checking that the animals are securely guarded at night, and handling all business relationships with the Chinese sponsor. It never works like that. The Chinese sponsor does not comprehend why it is that these pleasant, clever, but still obviously fishy animals should require food of a higher standard than he and his family purchase from the market, and water a hundred times clearer and purer than that in the sewage-contaminated river or canal nearby. Electricity and salt by the hundredweight and chlorine liquid and filter pumps with efficient motors all cost good money. Surely all that is really needed is a pool containing some water? These other things must be extravagances. As for the two days' rest after the journey from Europe before beginning performances, what nonsense! There is money to be made, and if the dolphins are swimming about as they patently are, how can they possibly be tired? A few minutes' work every hour from eleven in the morning till ten at night could hardly be called unreasonable!

Thus a triangular situation is set up, the three corners being formed by the Chinese sponsor and the indefinite number of sub-sponsors behind him, the German agent's representative, and the dolphin trainer. Only the trainer has the interests of the animals at heart. But to whom can he turn when he urgently requires a bucket of this or a spare part for that? Who can he hold responsible if one day there are no fish for the dolphins?

First he goes to the agent's representative with his troubles. "Well, my dear boy," says the representative, "fish is supplied by the sponsor. I'll see him about it, but it really is his responsibility." Two days later, if nothing has happened, the trainer may find himself desperately confronting the impassive Chinese sponsor, if he can find him. Having found him he soon finds things becoming much more complicated. The sponsor either can't or doesn't want to understand what it's all about, or if he speaks some English will take this tack. "We agreed to buy a certain quantity of fish each week, and this has been written into our contract with the German agent. It seems that for one reason or another your animals have eaten more than I and my partners are due to pay for. Please go and tell the agent's representative that if you require more fish he must purchase it." When this bit of information is duly passed back to the agent, he of course denies the facts of the matter, and it all ends up either with the dolphins going hungry or the trainer having to pay for the food himself. A day's diet for two dolphins, twenty to thirty pounds of fish, can be quite expensive in many parts of the Far East, and the trainer, who is paid weekly by the representative, is rarely bursting with cash.

The difficulty of pinning down exactly who is going to pay for what becomes acute for the trainer when an expensive item of equipment is urgently required—as, for example, when a motor burns out and has to be replaced or when a new plastic liner is needed to replace one that is ripped or punctured. It is accepted that such things were to

be provided by the sponsor. He made the agreement with
the agent. But he cannot foot the bill alone; he will have to
approach the people to whom he sold parts of the deal,
and they must pay their share. The sub-sponsors in turn try
to lay off some of the expense on the sub-sub-sponsors. If
only one of them objects to stumping up his portion, the
others may refuse to put in their contribution.

The result is that the whole intricate network of responsibility and liability fouls up hopelessly. No one will
pay more than his share, so no one pays anything at all, and
the pump remains out of action or the pool continues to
leak, wasting vast quantities of water and salt, thereby producing another crop of disputes over who pays what.

There are only two losers: the pair of trusting cetaceans that uncomplainingly continue to swim in broth-like
water and wait for someone to pay their wages in handfuls
of sardine or butter fish.

Finally, in desperation, the trainer appeals to the dolphins' owner, and that is how Andrew and I often come to
be flying at a moment's notice to Jakarta or Taipei to try
to pick up the pieces of yet another animal tragedy, or
once in a while to try to prevent it. Most owners of dolphins have either heard or learned the hard way about the
folly of sending animals to the Far East. They are never
bitten twice. But occasionally we still come across in-
stances of a zoo or marineland that naïvely succumbs to the
promises of rich rewards with cast-iron guarantees of
high-standard conditions if they will send dolphins on the
well-worn show-business circuits around the South China
Sea.

Always in the Far East I find the difficulties of a purely
medical character which one faces in underdeveloped
tropical countries are complicated by extraneous political,
social, and economic factors. Dealing with these requires

more than just veterinary knowledge. On one occasion I had to wrangle with Chinese entrepreneurs who wanted to save electricity by turning off the big fans that cooled the air in a Singapore stadium. I was not concerned for the audiences, who had to endure the stifling humidity for only three quarters of an hour, but I was anxious about the water temperature of the dolphin pool. It was rising steadily towards the danger point above which the creatures might have difficulty in dispersing their excess body heat. The negotiations were difficult and carried out through an interpreter. It was important not to lose my temper or cause them to lose face. After hours of almost surrealistic exchanges over a matter which to any animal man is painfully obvious, they conceded the point. The fans would be started again.

"What impressed them about you, Dr. Taylor," said the interpreter afterwards, "was that you are rich and must therefore be someone to be respected as knowing his business."

"Rich!" I exclaimed. "Why on earth should they get that idea?" I was hardly well dressed and was sporting no gold teeth or expensive jewellery.

"Your tummy," replied the interpreter, tapping the results of too much car driving and sitting in aircraft seats. "You are getting a belly, they said, the sign of the prosperous one." (Shelagh hadn't said anything about prosperity when she had recently reproved me about incipient broadening of my waistline.)

The following year I was in Sumatra, dealing with skin disease caused by filthy water when the sponsors had refused to mend a filter pump. A few months later I was called to Bandung in the hill country of Java: A dolphin was seriously ill and there were big problems. I flew out to Jakarta and was met by a representative of the German agents. He had not received the telegram giving my arrival time but had sat on at the airport for three days and met every passenger disembarking with "Dr. Taylor, yes?" He whipped me through customs and immigration and took me to a car. "Only a four-hour drive to Bandung," he said.

I was very tired by my long jet flight and wondered what it must have been like for the poor dolphins. After being unloaded from the aircraft they too must have set off by this road, but in a wagon which would have taken far longer than four hours.

I am not sure what my companion was thinking or to which branch of the show-biz fraternity I belonged when he said, "Before we go any further, Doctor, I should warn you that all artistes who have come to Java up to this time, without exception, have caught VD."

"Oh, thank you very much," I murmured.

We passed over a wooden bridge spanning a shallow wooded valley. Below in the stream a young woman with long gleaming black hair and a green and red batik sarong paddled naked from the waist upwards. It was a warm, scented evening with a sky of fluorescent salmon pink. We bounced along, climbing steadily through hills neatly stepped with paddy fields and crusted with dense green tea plantations. Then we slipped over the range and dropped down into Bandung, a bustling, friendly city, full of colour and the babble of voices, of old Dutch colonial villas, neat little houses covered with lush tropical vegetation, higgledy-piggledy conglomerations of shanties, temples, and colourful bird markets, and swarms of rickshaws.

I went straight to the dolphins, in one of the poorer quarters. A simple pair of portable plastic swimming pools stood in the middle of an arena made from wooden laths and partly roofed with palm leaves. The water was brown and contained a high concentration of particles; it looked for all the world like oxtail soup but smelled like rotten fish. Juan, the dolphin trainer, an old friend from England, was in a terrible state over his animals. One was very ill and losing weight by the hour, and to cap it all the Chinese sponsors had cut up rough. Sick dolphin, they had said, meant no show. No show meant no people. No people meant they were not going to pay money for electricity or water or salt or food. Two people had been killed the day before in the crush trying to get into the arena to see Flipper. Now the police were on guard outside.

In my usual tropical kit, my underpants, I jumped into the pool to examine the sick dolphin, Rocky. He was in a bad way, with thin, diseased skin and half-closed, lethargic eyes. I went over him carefully and found an enlarged liver lobe bulging back beyond the last rib, which suggested liver disease.

When working in the East I rarely have problems getting blood samples processed, since there is usually a mission hospital or similar institution with a lab only too willing to help out in an emergency. Sure enough, within half an hour I had located an American Pentecostal hospital that readily agreed to analyse a blood sample from Rocky. A couple of hours later the results came back. It was hepatitis. The dolphin was in danger of complete liver collapse and death within a very short space of time.

I went back to the pool and opened the bag of tricks that I always carry with me. I had little doubt that the infection had come from the foul water, though the fish that were being fed to the dolphins looked none too wholesome either. It would take a few days to identify exactly the bacterium responsible, and by then Rocky might be dead. I decided to assume that the germ causing the liver infection was one of a group which often affects dolphins; a fre-

quenter of water and bad fish, it is totally resistant to penicillin and most antibiotics. I would have to use a drug rarely
employed at the time in treating animals in Britain, the
highly efficient gentamicin.

Experimenting years before at Flamingo Park, I had
found that because dolphin kidneys are more efficient at
throwing the stuff off, three times the dose for a human
being of equivalent weight was needed to achieve a curative
level of gentamicin in the dolphin bloodstream. At this rate
it would cost around £60 a day for Rocky's antibiotic alone.
I would also have to give him drugs to aid the weakening
liver cells and replace chemicals that the organ was too
weak to manufacture. Also, it is no good giving gentamicin
by mouth, as it just is not absorbed from the bowel. Rocky
would need to be injected four times a day.

So began an intensive course of treatment to clear the
dolphin's system of the poisons building up because of the
liver failure. He was unable to take part in any performances and Flipper, his mate, was unwilling to do any tricks
without him. The management was extremely annoyed; it
was most unco-operative and inconsiderate of the animal to
fall ill. What about the paying customers, who would give
their right arms to get in? And why, now that the dolphin
doctor from England had given the animal the once-over
and an injection of golden liquid, wasn't the wretched
Rocky hard at it again? Hadn't he heard? The show must
go on!

A compromise of sorts had to be reached. I insisted
that Rocky had to rest; the sponsors wanted to put on a
show and make rupiahs. So it came about that the public
was admitted four times a day to watch an extraordinary
kind of dolphin show.

When all the customers were packed into the rows of
seats around the pool, the compère would do his usual

warm-up introduction to the amazing "lumba-lumbas," as the dolphins are called in Indonesian. He would explain that Rocky was a bit off-colour so Flipper would not do his stuff very well, but, he would add, he had a special treat for the crowd.

At great expense, all the way from England, the management has brought the unique, the amazing, the incredible per-for-ming dolphin doctor! Applause from the audience.

For the first time ever in Asia, complete with hypodermic needle and stethoscope, Dr. David Taylor will examine and inject the sick Rocky! At this point ninety-five per cent of the audience are standing on their seats for a better view.

*And now to introduce the man who knows all the secrets of a lumba-lumba's sex life—*the tape recording of "A Life on the Ocean Wave" is turned up to maximum volume—*your friend and mine, Dr. Taylor from Lancashire, England!*

Out from the fish-kitchen I walk in my underpants. The members of the audience grin, cheer, and applaud enthusiastically. With a great show of net-twirling, Juan and his assistants catch the torpid dolphin. I bow to the crowd, wave my stethoscope in the air, then get down to the serious business of giving Rocky his essential treatment. When it comes to the filling of the syringe with the gentamicin I hold up the bottles so that the audience can see every detail of the process. The empty vials are eagerly sought after by small boys in the front row. There is a great *a-a-a-ah* from the crowd as I insert the needle and more clapping as I withdraw it and rub the site with an antiseptic swab.

Four times a day I trod the boards, and by the end of the week Rocky was coming back strongly and the sponsors had coined a small fortune. The trouble was that the fortune was not big enough, nowhere near what they had hoped for. A few days after I began my act I had bigger trouble than ever. The leader of the syndicate came to the arena one evening and personally removed all the electrical power fuses, venting his anger with the agent on the innocent dolphins. Without an amp of electricity in the place their water was totally unfiltered, there were no lights for my night injections, and the fish in the refrigerator were rapidly going bad. I was livid. The sponsor had gone into a deep huff and refused to see Juan or the representative of the German agent. Flipper and Rocky cruised round in even thicker oxtail soup. I put a ban on feeding the putrefying fish and went to see the sponsor. Whether he liked it or not, I would sit on his doorstep until I had words with him.

Eventually I was let in and invited to talk with him. "I bear you personally no ill-will," he said, "but these animals that cannot work are causing me much anguish. It is not just money, it is a political problem. You see, we Chinese in countries like Indonesia have to be very careful. There are racial tensions here, although you may not sense it at the moment. Last year a Chinese sponsor promoted a show in Bandung and something went wrong, he didn't give the people what he'd promised, and it sparked off an explosion of resentment among the native Indonesian majority. They took it out on all the Chinese community, not just the sponsor. Cars of Chinese had their windscreens broken and tyres slashed. Some houses were set on fire. It could easily happen again. Chinese businessmen in the Far East are widely resented by other races in the community. I really believe we Chinese sit on a tinder-box. So if the dolphin show that I promote this year is regarded as a wash-out and doesn't come up to the Indonesians' expectations, I could have big trouble, and so could all the other Chinese in Bandung. That is why we don't use banks for our savings but hoard little gold ingots. You can never tell what will happen tomorrow."

So it was yet another political affair involving dolphins. "But you must see my point of view also," I replied. "I am here solely to look after the health of the dolphins. The sooner Rocky is OK, the sooner the show can be a big hit."

The Chinaman nodded impassively and returned to his theme of racial tension. "Three days ago two people were killed, you know, trying to get into the show. How many next time? And suppose they blame it on me? I'd be crucified."

On and on we wrangled, but I made no headway. He was not going to spend money on keeping the dolphins unless they worked. In desperation I tried a different tack.

"Right, then," I said, standing up to go. "As you can do nothing for the animals, I personally must pay for the replacement of the fuses and for the water and electricity bills. The animals are not my property. I have no interest in the show. I am not an employee of the German agent or a shareholder in your syndicate. But we British are at least humane and civilized enough to protect the weak and inno-cent"—I hoped he had not heard of our fine English stag and otter hunters and the hare-coursing fraternity—"and, though I cannot afford it, I cannot see the dolphins die. Good evening."

I walked smartly towards the door. As I reached it, to my astounded delight he called me back. "Dr. Taylor," he said, "I have no quarrel with you. I will make inquiries to see who removed the fuses. The electricity will be on within the hour."

Good Lord, I thought, it really has worked. To avoid losing face he's suggesting that someone else turned off the power. Still, I had no wish to embarrass him and did not let on that I knew who had pulled the fuses.

"How very good of you!" I said, shaking his hand heartily. "I'll do my best to have Rocky in A-one shape as soon as possible." To improve things further I offered to mediate between him and the German agents and to thrash out a more reasonable arrangement for the rest of the tour.

Rocky recovered splendidly, and eventually he and Flipper came back to Europe for a well-earned rest. But they brought something back with them. From a batch of contaminated fish or a pool of unwholesome water in Asia they had picked up a virus. This evil little germ lay dormant in their bodies for many weeks, but in time it became active and began to multiply rapidly. Intensive efforts were made to destroy the germ, which like all viruses was resistant to antibiotics, but after a long period of illness both Rocky and Flipper died.

No one ever really escaped from Devil's Island.

13 Sharp Practice

OF ALL THE TRIPS ABROAD on which my work has taken
me, the one which may yet have the most far-reaching
results came about when, after years of fruitless applica-
tions for a visa to visit China, I was eventually invited in
1973 to spend two weeks studying animal acupuncture and
inspecting zoological collections in that country. At that
time few Western zoologists had been given the opportunity to see the Chinese animal collections, many of which
contain species never exhibited in the West. I was anxious
to see some of the rare creatures that inhabit China's most
inaccessible regions and to find out whether and to what
degree the science of acupuncture was being applied to animals, particularly undomesticated ones.

With Gary Smart, one of the directors of the Royal
Windsor Safari Park, I flew out to Peking. We arrived in
bitterly cold weather, and in the middle of the night, at
the forbidding, Stalinesque Peking airport, where we were
met by Mr. Lo, a delightful, slightly built young man who
was to be our guide, interpreter, and political mentor. He
told us we could go where we liked and photograph anything and explained that, although he had not handled a
veterinary scientist before, he had carefully prepared a
handwritten phrase book of words which might be needed

by him during our discourses. It was crammed with every
conceivable veterinary word from anaplasmosis to zonules
of Zinn, each with the corresponding Chinese ideogram.

"That, Dr. Taylor," he said, smiling broadly, "will
come in useful when we go round the zoos and hospitals.
But first, as a good friend of China, you will want to see
our progress in light engineering, agricultural communes,
heavy industry, textile production, and so forth."

We felt obliged to murmur our assent. For three days
we inspected light bulb factories and sheds where Peking
ducks were force-fed by machines. We were sung to by
infant schools and toured secondary schools where every
class had some special item of entertainment ready for us.
We looked at tractor exhibitions and blocks of flats, had
tea and sweets with little old ladies who told us how cruel
landlords used to be, and drank gallons of delightful green
tea with innumerable revolutionary committees, each member of which described a particular aspect of progress in
birth control, the manufacture of bricks, shipbuilding, or
the eradication of all traces of Confucianism. But not a
zoo, not a wolf or a snake, not a monkey or a panda did
we see.

We became increasingly anxious, fearing that the continuous socio-political hurly-burly might take up the
whole of our visit. Then began a series of visits to the great
and glorious relics of the old China: the Forbidden City,
the Great Wall, the Ming tombs and palaces, temples,
monasteries, and gardens. It was all immensely fascinating,
but still we saw no zoos.

Finally, our patience wearing if not thin at least somewhat slimmer, we felt that we had served our apprentice-
ship in Anglo-Chinese friendship and made forceful repre-
sentations to be shown the things that we had paid many
hundreds of pounds to come and see. At last we set foot
in our first Chinese zoo park, in Peking.

The zoo was stuffed with animals and birds that we had never seen before. There were giant Tibetan donkeys, the most dangerous animals in the zoo, we were told, when they are in the mating season. A north-east Chinese tiger far outstripped the record size given in the *Guinness Book of World Records*. There were reptiles and birds found only in remote corners of that vast country, and elephants and rhinoceroses only recently discovered in their own Chinese forests. We spent a long time admiring the fabulous golden monkeys from the snow-covered north. These unique primates with bright blue faces, snub noses, and long golden hair were the most handsome monkeys I have ever seen. Then there were the giant pandas, an adorable group of youngsters lying on their backs in the sun chewing sugar cane and bamboo.

All the animals seemed very healthy and contented, but when at the end of our tour of the zoo we had the usual formal meeting with the revolutionary committee that runs it, I could find out little about their veterinary services. They declined to show us the veterinary laboratory as being unworthy and inadequate, and they said that acupuncture was never used on the zoo stock. I asked for stool samples from the giant pandas, which I was keen to examine for parasites; there was always the chance that one would find some new and unnamed species of worm or fluke in the droppings of so rare a creature. Plastic bags full of droppings from each of the pandas were promptly produced. At the end of my visit I carefully carried them back to England, only to find on detailed microscopical examination that not one of the samples contained any sign of a single unwanted guest. My daydreams of being remembered by posterity through some obscure maggot bearing my latinized name were dashed.

After Peking we visited Shanghai and Canton zoos. At each the picture was the same—a priceless stock of mainly

Chinese animals, a polite but firm refusal to give information on medical care, and a complete lack of interest in buying from or exchanging animals with the West. As for selling animals to European zoos, it was politely explained that as the stock belonged to the people only the people could give permission. It was not altogether clear how the people went about voicing their opinions. No one cared to comment on the pandas given to certain Western heads of state or on the sensible exchanges of animals which had recently taken place with Whipsnade Zoo in England.

I was determined to see acupuncture being practised and insisted that Mr. Lo should organize it, since I was being frustrated in the primary aim of my Chinese trip. So we were taken to see it being done on humans. First we were shown dental clinics where patients sat in long rows of chairs receiving routine attention to their mouths. Some had opted for what we would call orthodox local anaesthetic injections to numb the pain. Others were receiving treatment under acupuncture anaesthesia, and these patients had one or two fine stainless-steel wires protruding from their hands or arms. Next we were taken to an outpatients' clinic where minor ailments such as headache, lumbago, and muscle sprains were being dealt with. In a small room we found a crowd of people of both sexes standing, sitting, or lying on benches. They positively sprouted needles all over the place, from heads, necks, arms, backs, legs, and toes. Not a drop of blood could be seen oozing anywhere. Later I saw a baby delivered and a lung lobe removed using the same techniques. In each case the patient was conscious and able to talk with the surgeons during the operation. But I still had to see acupuncture used on animals.

One day Mr. Lo arrived at our hotel to say that I was invited to the Central Veterinary Clinic in Peking, where an operation had been laid on. We drove out to the clinic, a complex of single-storey buildings covered with anti-revisionist slogans. The revolutionary committee of veterinarians welcomed us with the usual tea-party and hour of political instruction before we got down to business. It was explained that although they used acupuncture anaesthesia in around two hundred major operations on cattle, horses, and mules each year, they had not got any large animal needing surgery on the day of my visit. To my dismay, although I must admit I felt unwilling to try to stop them, they proposed to operate on a perfectly healthy old horse and remove a piece of its large intestine.

First they gave me a carefully prepared lecture, illustrated with pictures pinned up on the wall, on the precise anatomical landmarks used for finding the correct acupuncture spot for each operation. It appeared that the clinic was using the method as a matter of routine for surgery of the head, chest, and abdomen, although they reported only fair results in removing sensation from the limbs below the elbow or knee. Research, they said, was continuing into animal acupuncture anaesthesia; the operation that I would see that day would require only two needles, whereas a year before they would have had to use fourteen for the same job. Research and refinement of the technique for locating the needle points precisely by using a sort of galvanometer that detects changes in the electrical resistance of the skin at these points, together with the diligent application of Chairman Mao's thoughts, had rendered twelve needles redundant.

We went into a rather odd operating theatre that resembled a Pennine cow byre and all donned white gowns, caps, and masks. The place was poorly equipped and badly in need of painting but they did have a useful-looking, hydraulically operated large-animal operating table. A tired

old grey mare was led in and hobbled to the table in the
vertical position and, when secure, gently revolved until
she was lying on her side. A woman anaesthetist produced
two long acupuncture needles which had been sterilizing in
a pan boiling away on a gas ring and indicated the points
which had been described in my briefing. For complete
anaesthesia of the left side of the horse's abdomen and
bowels she was going to put one needle into the left foreleg above the knee and the other into the same leg but
below the knee. Swabbing the chosen sites with alcohol,
she inserted the needles. The one above the knee was
pressed diagonally downwards through the flesh until it
had almost transfixed the limb and was tenting the skin on
the inside of the leg.

Mr. Lo moaned as he stood beside me. "Dr. Taylor,
I am going to be sick," he said, turning away. He was certainly going green above his mask.

For the mare the insertion of the needle was probably
no more painful than having a deep shot of local anaesthetic, and she lay calmly enough. When the needles were
exactly in position, wires from an alternating current generator were clipped to them. Knobs were turned and dials
were set on the machine. Small muscles in the leg near the
acupuncture needles began to twitch and flicker.

"Now we wait for ten minutes," said the anaesthetist.
"Then the surgeon can begin."

Ten minutes passed. The horse lay blinking and sup-
ping water through a tube from a kettle. The foreleg
muscles continued to twitch, but otherwise there was nothing to suggest that the animal was anything but totally
conscious. The surgeon picked up his scalpel.

I clenched my fists under my gown. He was going to
have to open the flank for a good twelve inches in one
continuous incision biting deep through skin and fat. Rather

you than me, old boy, I thought. It was impossible to believe that those two needles and the electric box buzzing away by the horse's head could have removed all feeling of pain from an apparently unrelated area several feet away. Nothing I had learned in those long days at university in Glasgow, taking formaldehyde-pickled horse corpses to bits under the eagle eyes of the anatomy tutor, had suggested any link between the foreleg and the belly. I was a prisoner of my Western training. What do we really know about the nervous system, particularly the elusive network that we call the autonomic? I was to come to believe that it was in this microscopic infrastructure of communication and command that the secret of acupuncture lay.

The scalpel pressed down onto the flesh and with a single elegant stroke the horse's side was unzipped down to the muscle layers. The animal did not bat an eyelid. I was watching intently for any sign of tensing or other reaction to the sudden pain of the knife, but there was nothing. The surgeon deftly opened the muscle, then sliced through the most sensitive layer of all, the peritoneum. A horse's peritoneum is thick and packed with nerve endings. Surely now the old grey would wince or struggle? No, she just supped on at her kettle.

The loops of intestine were now visible. The surgeon pulled gently and then vigorously on a loop. Oddly enough the bowel and its attachments have no nerve endings that can detect cutting or even burning, but they do contain lots of endings that scream blue murder at the slightest tugging, stretching, or twisting. That is why horses suffer such pain from the griping distensions and distortions of the bowel in colic, pain that can literally shock them to death. This old grey seemed totally oblivious to the pulling.

Expertly the surgeon took out a portion of the bowel

wall and stitched up the incision; then smoothly and rapidly he closed the various layers of the operation wound. Half an hour later the skin was closed. The anaesthetist switched off the electric machine and withdrew the needles. The table was returned to an upright position and the old horse was released. Steady as a rock, and dropping a healthy pile of manure on the way, she walked outside into the yard and began to eat corn heartily from a trough. I was most impressed.

Over the next few days I spent as much time as I could with the vets at the clinic. They had no experience of working with zoo animals, and as dogs and cats are regarded as unproductive creatures and are rarely seen in China (they are as rare as flies, which have been almost completely eradicated; during two weeks in the country we saw no dogs, one cat, and two flies), they could give no advice about using acupuncture on carnivores. However, charts of the acupuncture points on horses, cattle, and humans, together with sets of needles and even little plastic men and animals on which to practise, are widely and cheaply available throughout China. The man in the street and the "barefoot doctors," the medical auxiliary workers who go into the countryside to take medical attention to the peasants and the peasants' animals, are encouraged to become proficient in this cheap and highly portable means of wide-ranging therapy.

China convinced me that there is a place in Western medicine for the development of acupuncture. If I worked with small animals such as dogs and cats I would experiment with the needles on certain conditions which are still difficult to tackle thoroughly by orthodox methods. Nervous diseases, fits, paralysis, arthritic conditions, and skin diseases seem ideal areas for investigation. But how to use the technique on my patients, the zoo animals?

By studying the charts of the cow and the horse and the man which I had brought back from China, together with a set of "barefoot doctor" needles and a small electric machine, I realized that the needle insertion point which treats a specific type of disease or produces anaesthesia of a particular area is in the same corresponding anatomical position in each of the three species. For example, the point on the human hand between the base of the thumb and the index finger, which affects the teeth, is anatomically identical to the position on the outside of the cow's foot or on top of the horse's cannon bone which affects the teeth in those species. In difficult cases which were not yielding to conventional treatment, I would try transposing the acupuncture points of the horse, cow, or man onto my zoo patients. It would be difficult with uniquely shaped animals like dolphins, and I have since learned that American vets have so far had no luck in identifying the acupuncture areas in these creatures. Still, the striking improvement in many cases of dolphin disease where the animal has been pricked with injection needles carrying perhaps only vitamin shots suggests that it is not always the medication that does the trick but that unwittingly the hypodermics may have hit the bull's-eye on an acupuncture point.

Shortly after returning from China I had my first suitable case for acupuncture. Eddie, a young giraffe at Royal Windsor Safari Park, had been dogged with chronic recurring arthritis of all four ankle joints ever since he had damaged the joints repeatedly during a rough passage through the Bay of Biscay on his way to Britain as a baby. Eddie's joints were a mess—enlarged, thickened with scar tissue round the joint capsule, and prone to flare up frequently into a painful, laming, inflammatory condition. He had had all sorts of treatment, from poultices and cortisone to courses of gold and new anti-arthritic drugs. Nothing worked for long. I decided to give Eddie five twenty-minute courses of acupuncture at weekly intervals, using points on his body that were anatomically equivalent to the ones which the Chinese used for polyarthritis in cattle.

Eddie was enticed by succulent oak branches into a restraining pen where he was unable to turn round or back away. With the aid of a ladder I climbed up the side of the pen and selected the two points over the rib-cage which I hoped would do the trick. I disinfected the skin and pushed the thin needles in about one inch deep. Eddie did not seem to care; he was used to injections, and these needles were far finer than the ones used for administering drugs. I clipped on the two wires leading to the generator, which was powered by a tiny transistor radio battery. Tense with anticipation I turned on the control switch. A little red light began to flash in the box. I adjusted the frequency control according to the instructions I had received in China, and the superficial muscles in the skin between the two needles began to twitch. Eddie continued to munch oak leaves. Twenty minutes later I switched off, withdrew the needles, and climbed down the ladder. Eddie limped away.

The giraffe's condition appeared unchanged, but three days later the giraffe keeper reported a definite improvement in Eddie's gait. I was not prepared even to hope that it was because of the acupuncture, but one week later I repeated the treatment. Eddie was undoubtedly walking much better, and I had a sneaking suspicion that his joints were not quite so grotesquely enlarged. The next week I was certain. Eddie's joints were on the mend.

By the time the course of treatments was complete the giraffe's joints were almost down to normal size, better than we had ever seen them since he had arrived, and he walked gracefully without a trace of a limp. Now the question was whether the arthritis would relapse after a time just as it had done following all the other forms of therapy. We waited. One, two, three weeks went by. Two months passed and still Eddie's joints were holding up. He had never been sound for so long. After four months we decided that it was fair to claim that he had made a remarkable recovery quite different from the temporary improvements seen in the past.

It left me itching to try the technique on some more knotty cases in exotic animals, but my second acupuncture patient turned out to be my elder daughter, Stephanie. Going home one evening I found her miserable with a toothache. Remembering the dental clinic I had seen in China and the ease with which the acupuncturists had numbed the teeth via a readily locatable point on the hand, I prevailed upon her to let me use my magic box and needle on her. Reluctantly, but remembering my frequent enthusiastic progress reports on Eddie, she agreed. Two minutes after I had popped in the needle she announced that the toothache had gone. Whatever the explanation of the mechanism behind acupuncture, I admit that in her case suggestion may have played an important part. But when I see Eddie cantering in the sunlight with that fluid motion so charming and so typical of giraffes, his ankles slim and free from ugly knobbles, I am certain that nobody suggested anything to him.

14 The Dying Unicorns

WORK WITH ZOO ANIMALS always has been very much feast or famine. For days I can sit in my office with very few, if any, calls coming in. I begin to wonder whether the telephone will ever ring again, my spirits get lower, and it seems as if the bottom has dropped out of my speciality. Turning down the regular four or five calls for domestic animals which we still receive even so many years after leaving general practice begins to seem increasingly pointless. But it does give me time to catch up with my reading in the journals on zoo animal affairs, and I can spend some time with Shelagh and the children.

At other times I am rushed off my feet and there seems to be enough work for half a dozen vets. The trouble is that there is no pattern to the incidence of exotic disease. Whereas a vet in small-animal practice has certain peaks and troughs in his work schedule, and a large-animal vet knows that lambings and cases of grass staggers and erysipelas will occur in well-defined periods, for me every day of the year is the same—unpredictable.

One grey, drizzly breakfast-time in November during a particularly dull spell the telephone rang. It was the

Director of Medical Services in Qatar, Dr. Gotting.
Sheikh Qassim's oryx were dying like flies. Could I go at
once to see what was up? A first-class ticket on the next
flight to the Arabian Gulf would be waiting for me at
London Airport.

The tall and elegant Arabian oryx is the most beautiful of all the antelopes: a dazzling creamy colour, with
crisp brown face and leg markings, its head topped with a
pair of long, tapering, backward-pointing horns. So sym-
metrically are the two horns set on its head that viewed
from the side it appears to have only one; it is probably
the animal men have mistaken for the mythical unicorn.
Beneath the handsome exterior, its anatomy and physiology
have evolved over the millennia into an amazing organism
capable of living and reproducing in one of the world's
most terrible deserts, the Empty Quarter of Arabia.

With ingenious internal tricks to cope with the shortage of natural water and to stop its blood from rising to
boiling point in the searing heat, with finely tuned senses
that can detect danger at great distances or locate springs
of water under the sand, and with the ability to outrun all
but the fastest carnivores, the Arabian oryx once pros-
pered. Then came the hunters. It was a strong and brave
collector of skin and horn who could penetrate the fastnesses of the oryx, and at first, because of the risk and
effort involved, the number of animals killed was not excessive. But when Arab sheikhs with big air-conditioned
Chevrolets and sub-machine-guns took to hunting, the
death warrant for this wild, beautiful animal was sealed.
They were slaughtered as trophies until, it is believed, not
one remains in the wild free state.

At least the species is not yet truly extinct, for Sheikh
Qassim had captured a number of the oryx and set up a
precious breeding herd on his desert farm. Another small

herd was established at Phoenix Zoo, Arizona, and odd animals can be found in a very few other zoos, but the total number of Arabian oryx alive today is fewer than one hundred.

Later that day I flew out to Doha, the capital of Qatar. When we landed in the early hours of the morning the scene on the tarmac was like something out of *The Seven Pillars of Wisdom*. Arabs in black robes and white turbans, carrying rifles and automatic machine-guns and with bandoliers of gleaming bullets criss-crossing their chests, clustered round the bottom of the steps. At first I thought they were there for me, but then I saw that they were exchanging greetings with a small Arab gentleman in traditional dress who had preceded me down the gangway. Later I found out that he was the very man whose oryx I had come to examine, Sheikh Qassim, and that the armed men were his personal bodyguard.

Dr. Gotting and Dr. Qayyum, who was the Chief Veterinary Officer, made up my welcoming party. With the minimum of formalities I was whisked through customs and immigration and taken to a hotel. I was impressed by the speed and efficiency; they certainly were not wasting any time. Over a cup of camomile tea I asked Dr. Qayyum about the outbreak of disease in the oryx. I was anxious to begin work as soon as dawn broke, and any history learned now would save valuable time.

"When was the last death, how many have died, and do you have any fresh post-mortem material for me?" I asked.

Dr. Qayyum looked a little embarrassed. "Twelve animals died," he replied, "but I'm afraid we have no post-mortem material."

"But when was the last death? Are any others likely to die in the next day or two?"

"The last death, Dr. Taylor, was in April, but on exactly which date in April I cannot recall."

I was flabbergasted. It was now the middle of November; the last deaths in this apparent emergency had occurred over six months before.

"But I believe you are having serious problems with the oryx," I said after I had regained my composure. "Are any ill at all at present?"

Qayyum shrugged his shoulders and made a despairing grimace. "I am not sure," he said, "but His Excellency the Sheikh is very worried about them. That is why he has returned today from London where he has been himself for treatment. He is very, very fond of the animals. He says no more must die."

"So you have no post-mortem reports or specimens from the last deaths?"

"Well, no. But we opened one or two."

"What did you find in those, Dr. Qayyum?"

"Nothing much. Perhaps the lungs were redder than normal."

"And you have no preserved specimens?"

He shook his head sadly.

"Well, how many oryx are left now?" I asked.

Dr. Qayyum shrugged again. "I do not know exactly, but tomorrow if you wish you can go to see them with my assistant, Dr. Iftikhar. Then you can see exactly how many there are."

At daybreak the following morning I set out from the hotel with Dr. Iftikhar, a smartly dressed young Pakistani who had recently arrived in Qatar. Doha is a small town of dusty buildings set on the water's edge, backed by desert which rolls away into the vast Empty Quarter, the Rub' al Khali. Graceful dhows lie in the harbour side by side with modern steamships carrying fertilizer and chicken feed for the embryo livestock industry. There are opulent palaces surrounded by trees and elegant pierced walls, and a modern, cool, emerald-green mosque. Women in black veils, their faces hidden behind beaked black-gold masks, ride by in Lincoln Continentals, and knots of men squat at street corners inspecting trussed hunting hawks. There are dim, bustling souks filled with the tinsmith's wares, vegetables, sherbet, spices, and Kraft margarine. The dust swirls in the streets as diggers and excavators work to build this new city out of the rocky desert. The inescapable sound of Radio Cairo is everywhere, carried by the ubiquitous transistor radio.

We drove out into the desert, a flat khaki plain covered by rocks and rubble for as far as the eye could see. Small grey-green tufts of wiry shrubbery somehow survive in places, and on these the nomadic shepherds graze their flocks of sheep and goats. On and on we travelled across the depressing flatland until a small oasis of trees came into view. As we got nearer I could see that a cluster of farm buildings and paddocks was set beneath the trees. Nearby was a small unpretentious palace. This was Al Zubarrah, Sheikh Qassim's weekend retreat, from where he keeps in touch with events in the capital by radio telephone. A tall radio antenna was fixed to the roof of the little mosque within the palace garden. A man sleeping on the ground in the shade of a windowless one-room hut by the gate of a large paddock awoke as we rumbled up and came forward to greet us. Dr. Iftikhar introduced him as the man who looked after the oryx.

The paddocks were built on the desert sand with high walls of grey breeze blocks and wide wooden doors. It was impossible to see what was inside them. Dense clouds of pigeons wheeled overhead and the entire area was littered with rubbish and crusted with birds' droppings. Even so, I was excited; few European zoologists had been to see Sheikh Qassim's farm. Within a few moments I would see for the first time the largest existing herd of an animal rarer than the giant panda or the komodo dragon. The oryx keeper took us over to the paddock gate, struggled with a rusty lock, and pushed open the heavy doors. We walked through into a sunlit compound which had a line of green trees planted all along one side.

Standing glowing in the morning sun at the far end of the paddock, heads turned in our direction, were the oryx, each one motionless and alert with ears pricked and nostrils distended. Quietly we walked towards them across the sand. There were troughs of sparkling fresh water, barley, and some sort of rough salt supplement set out under the trees. Piles of lush, freshly cut lucerne lay on the ground nearby. The oryx certainly seemed to be fed and watered carefully. As we came within fifty yards of the herd they moved off, circling round us close to the grey walls. What gorgeous creatures they were! Beige-coloured calves pressed next to cantering adults with flanks of dazzling whiteness and horns as straight and even and shiny as rapiers.

There were thirty-three animals, and all of them looked in tip-top condition, plump and well-rounded. Only one elderly female had a hygroma, a sac of fluid the size of a grapefruit (a sort of chronic housemaid's knee) on one knee joint.

"They look very healthy, Dr. Iftikhar," I said. "Do they breed well?"

"We get six or eight calves each year," he replied. "The herd size increases quite rapidly, but then disease seems to strike and we're down to around thirty again."

Questioning him in detail about the last deaths in April produced little of importance. There was not much to go

on, just the vaguest of histories. Whatever it was that was
killing the oryx, it struck suddenly as a rapidly fatal epi-
demic and then apparently disappeared when the numbers
of oryx had been trimmed back. This pattern suggested
that overcrowding and population density might be important factors. But suppose one day the disease just went
on spreading through the herd until it wiped out the lot
or at least a minimum breeding group? It was a frightening
thought.

While I stood and watched the oryx and they circled
warily round us, there was a commotion in the air above
us as a flock of pigeons numbering about two thousand
swept over the wall of the oryx paddock and descended
on the troughs of barley. The oryx keeper chased them
away and they rose in a noisy, dusty blue-black cloud.

"I've never seen so many pigeons in my life," I remarked. "Why does the Sheikh keep so many?"

"To feed and train his falcons," was the reply. "After
the oryx, Sheikh Qassim's greatest love is to hunt the
houbara."

The houbara is a fast-flying species of bustard living
in the desert. Rich Arab falconers take fleets of air-conditioned cars, dozens of trained hawks and falcons, and a
retinue of staff into the Rub' al Khali for one or two weeks
at a time and are perfectly satisfied if they return with just
one houbara.

Dr. Iftikhar showed me round the rest of the farm.
As we went out of the gate of the oryx paddock, a group
of camels were ambling by. Their coats were sparse and
the underlying skin was an unhealthy crusty pink. They
were extensively affected by mange. Whenever they got the
chance they would stop against the corner of a wall or the
trunk of a tree and have a satisfying rub. Mange is common
in camels and it makes them itch, but the rubbing helps

to spread the disease. Dr. Iftikhar explained that the camels were passing through the farm. The nomad herdsmen used the farm as a stopping place and every day one or two herds of camel or sheep would rest there, taking advantage of the water and shade for an hour or two while the herdsmen exchanged gossip and took a cup of tea with the Sheikh's men.

We entered another paddock, but this one contained only seven minute Arabian gazelles, which leaped about in panic as we opened the gate. Iftikhar explained that the Sheikh had collected these also. Originally there had been nearly eighty but the disease had hit them, too. Again, there were no post-mortem examination reports or preserved specimens.

A third paddock contained sheep and goats. Conditions there were markedly different from the oryx enclosure. The animals were thin and in poor condition. Their food troughs were empty. Many had infected eyes, purulent noses, and maggot-infested sores.

"These are a terribly poor lot, Dr. Iftikhar," I exclaimed, picking up a small, almost comatose lamb that lay dying in the fierce heat of midday. "Riddled with disease and half-starved, I'd say."

Dr. Iftikhar began a verbose apology. Yes, they were a problem. No, they didn't have enough food. Sadly, no one seemed to be able to do anything about them. But it was all the fault of a batch of sheep brought in from Saudi Arabia. You really couldn't trust the people over there to eradicate their diseases. He rattled on and took me by the arm, drawing me away from the miserable animals that were unusually silent, so weak and debilitated had they become.

"I'm sure you don't want to get yourself messed up with these creatures, Dr. Taylor." He brushed flecks of

wool and dirt from his natty suit. "After all, you are here
to see the oryx."

"I'm here to look into the oryx disease problem," I
said, more than a little disgruntled. "I may be six months
late, but at least I may find out something by knowing
what sort of sick animals the oryx have as their next-door
neighbours. Please arrange for this lamb to be killed now
so that I can do an autopsy on the spot."

I could see in Dr. Iftikhar's face that I was disturbing
the peace and order of his routine.

"But we have no facilities, Dr. Taylor. It is only a
lamb. Lambs die all the time."

"Of course they do, but they die from something. I
have all I need in my bag. Please get me a container of
water for my hands."

When the skinny little body of the lamb was brought
I crouched under the shade of a tree and made a crude
dissection. Dr. Iftikhar stood some yards off, watching.
The chest cavity was full of sticky, honey-coloured liquid. The tiny lungs were affected by dropsy and carried
large areas of solid purple inflammation. The lymph glands
draining the lungs were enlarged and angry-looking,
spotted with bright scarlet haemorrhages. It looked like
haemorrhagic septicaemia, a disease of cattle, buffalo,
sheep, and wild cud-chewing animals which is caused by
a bacterium called Pasteurella. I took specimens for analysis
and culture. If I could find Pasteurella in this lamb, perhaps
I could begin to explain the sudden deaths in the oryx
and gazelles. The teeming legions of foraging pigeons
would be the obvious carriers of the disease over the wall
to the oryx.

In the other farm buildings the earth floors were piled
high with mounds of long-dead birds: hens, turkey poults,
and pigeons. Emaciated hens stalked hungrily about, peck-

ing at the remains of their fellows that were slowly rotting
into the ground. Every room, cage, hut, and pen contained
dead or dying birds. Pigeons fluttered everywhere. Many
of them were sick, their eyes half closed and the skin of
the eyelids, at the corners of the mouth, and around the
nostrils distended with masses of warts and blisters. The
decaying corpses of turkeys and hens bore the same ugly
excrescences. Pox virus was rampant. I wondered what
Andrew, who has a special interest in bird diseases and has
published a paper on pox in falcons, would think of this
charnel-house. If Sheikh Qassim was feeding pigeons to his
valuable hunting birds, he must surely be suffering losses
from pox attacks.

The farm was literally stuffed with diseased animals.
Only the oryx and gazelles were in good condition, and
they alone showed any evidence of being systematically
fed. Carrying samples of the oryx food, including fresh and
dried lucerne, I was driven back across the seventy miles
of desert to Doha. Without dead or sick animals among
the oryx there was little I could do to confirm the nature
of the disease, but I was fairly certain that haemorrhagic
septicaemia was the culprit.

On the way back to the city Dr. Iftikhar asked me
to give my opinion on a case of lameness in a horse at Al
Rayyan, the royal stables. We drove up to an imposing
arrangement of white buildings. Round a vast sandy arena
were rows of spacious, airy loose-boxes. It was most im-
pressive. We stood in the sunlight as a groom led out a
chestnut Thoroughbred. It was thin and rangy and had a
pronounced limp in one foreleg. I examined the leg and Dr.
Iftikhar described the history and his course of treatment.
It was a case of navicular disease, inflammation of a peculiar but troublesome little bone that lies beneath the
horny wall of a horse's (or zebra's) hoof. When we had

agreed on a plan for further therapy I remarked on the poor condition of the animal. Dr. Iftikhar looked embarrassed once again.

"I'm afraid that the horses here have little food. There are sixty of them, blood horses from Britain, Ireland, and Germany. But they belong to the ex-Emir."

"What difference does that make?"

Dr. Iftikhar puffed and scratched his head. "Well, it's a peculiar business. The old Emir was deposed bloodlessly by the present ruler, his younger brother. Now he's in exile. But because it's something of a family affair, all his belongings in Qatar remain his property. The new Emir and the rest of the family won't confiscate them, but on the other hand they won't find any money to maintain them. It doesn't matter very much in the case of buildings or motorcars, but unfortunately there are more serious consequences for his horses."

"Do you mean that no one feeds the horses?"

"Well, sometimes they get a little, but not often."

"Why doesn't the government sell or destroy the horses?"

"Because they belong to the exiled Emir."

Iftikhar led the way into the well equipped looseboxes, in each of which was a horse. They were all obviously of first-quality breeding with fine heads and superb bones. There were greys and chestnuts, bays and blacks, but every one was in some stage of plain, down-to-earth starvation. Some stood like hatracks, their fine skin pulled tight over their skeletons; others lay unable to rise. Some chewed at the sandy floor. Their droppings were a mixture of sand, wood dust, and mucus. At least there was plenty of water but of any kind of food there was not a trace in the whole complex. I walked on past box after box, unable to believe my eyes. Animals that would be worth hundreds of thousands of pounds in Europe were being allowed to starve slowly to death. And I had been asked to look at a case of lameness!

"Doesn't all this eating of sand and earth produce gut trouble?" I asked, literally dizzy with disbelief. "Surely you get colic cases galore?"

"Yes, we do. That's what finishes them usually. I treat them with Pethidine if they're in pain."

It may have been a bloodless deposing of the old Emir, I thought, but it had meant a cruel death for a collection of innocent animals brought far from the pastures of their birth.

"Is there nothing we can do about it?" I asked.

"I'm afraid not," said Dr. Iftikhar. "It's very difficult to influence such matters. High politics, you know. Ruling family and so forth."

I would try to do something about it.

Back in my hotel I decided to go for a swim in the sea before changing my clothes for one of Sheikh Qassim's traditional audiences that evening. The waters of the Gulf behind the Alwaha Hotel were shallow, pale blue, and highly inviting. As I swam I could see large dark shadows scurrying about on the ocean bottom, but without goggles or a face mask I was unable to identify them. Then I saw an Arab wading about in the water carrying a large tin slung round his shoulders and peering through the water with the aid of an empty jam jar. From time to time he would dive quickly beneath the surface and come up with the biggest pink and brown crabs I had ever seen. So that's what the scurrying shadows were. I swam on, thinking how delectable they would be prepared in Shelagh's favourite way with the meat dressed with white wine, garlic, and capers and roasted in the shell. Suddenly the Arab gave a mighty yell, dropped his tin and his jam jar, and plunged off with great leaping strides towards the shore. I wondered if one of his quarry had laid hold of his foot, since the crabs were big enough to pinch severely.

Floating lazily on, I looked down through the clear water at the fuzzy shapes on the bottom and revelled in the cool caress of the sea. One of the dark shapes did not scurry like the others; in fact, it was not on the sea bottom at all. It grew bigger. It was swimming towards me, effortlessly and straight as an arrow. It had the strangest head and it was brown on top and dirty white underneath. Suddenly I knew what had made the crab-catcher head so rapidly for dry land, for coming lazily towards me was a full-grown hammerhead shark. The bizarre shape of the head, which is five times as wide as it is long, was unmistakable. The hammerhead is definitely known to be a man-eater. Certainly it is not fussy about what it eats; I had seen them take dead dolphins caught in the nets in Florida. I felt very, very frightened.

On came the hammerhead. Even underwater I could see him now with less distortion. I did not dare turn away from him to swim towards shore, nor did I fancy the idea of standing on the bottom with the water up to my chest. Then, when he was about six feet away, another of the busily hurrying crabs came teetering by. With its large, unblinking eyes the shark spotted the creature and suddenly veered off diagonally downwards. Through the shimmering water I saw it smoothly pick up the crab in its jaws. *Scrunch.* The crab disappeared. The hammerhead swirled round in the water, the tip of its tail flashed under my nose, and in a moment it had gone, gliding calmly away into deeper water. I made my way to the beach. I did not swim in the Gulf again.

At six o'clock it was time to go to one of the Sheikh's regular audiences, held twice a day at his town palace, or

Majlis. At these audiences anyone, from the highest to the lowest in the community, has a chance to exchange a few words with or make a request of the Sheikh. With Dr. Gotting I drove into the Majlis through an archway guarded by the armed men I had seen at the airport. Inside there were cool courtyards with fountains and orange trees, and cloisters where patient hawks sat hooded on their blocks.

We removed our shoes and entered a brightly lit room decorated with the heads of Arabian oryx mounted as trophies. At the far end on a decorated chair sat the Sheikh, and around him were seated members of the aristocracy and government ministers. The chair on his immediate right was empty. Here for short periods would sit those with whom he wished to talk or who had a petition to make. Down the sides of the room sat all sorts of other people, the least important and most shabbily dressed next to the door.

As we entered the Sheikh rose to greet us. The rest of the people in the room also stood. We walked the length of the room, shook hands, and retired to two seats halfway along the wall. Everyone took their seats once more. A little whispering was going on and the Sheikh would occasionally beckon to some member of his staff, who would come to sit briefly at the Sheikh's right and talk in low tones. A servant circulated continually with a tray of small handleless cups and an ornate gold pot full of camomile tea. My cup was kept permanently brimming, and I had to learn to shake the empty cup from left to right to indicate that I did not want any more of the rather insipid beverage.

It was a very leisurely business. Shabbily dressed peasants from near the door would seize their chance to sit in the vacant chair and then quickly murmur their request into the Sheikh's ear. Rarely was anyone there for more than a minute or two. If the Sheikh decided that action had to be taken, he would beckon to an official and give his instructions. Dr. Gotting explained that it was at just such an audience that Sheikh Qassim had suddenly become alarmed about the condition of the oryx and had commanded him to get professional help from Britain immediately. Although the good doctor supervised the running of the hospitals and was in no way involved with the veterinary services, he had had to take it in hand. The order might equally well have been given to the chief of police or the director of oil production. No matter who was given an order, he had to execute it.

After half an hour and an overabundance of tea, Dr. Gotting went to the chair and spoke with the Sheikh. When he returned he whispered to me that the Sheikh had asked him whether I had brought my family with me yet. Apparently he expected me to stay permanently!

"He thinks you are here for good to look after his oryx. He wasn't very pleased when I said you were only here on a short visit. He thinks you should remain ad infinitum."

Much as the Arabian oryx fascinated me, I could not conceive a worse fate than to spend all one's days out on that awful farm in the desert. A few minutes later the chair beside the Sheikh was empty again.

"Right, off you go now," whispered Dr. Gotting.

I went across to the chair and sat down. An interpreter came to stand behind the Sheikh.

"His Excellency asks what you think of the oryx at Al Zubarrah," he said.

I realized I would have to get my points over quickly and I wanted also to raise the matter of the horses starving at Al Rayyan.

"The oryx are very fine," I began, "but the cause of the disease cannot be precisely established yet. However, I do recommend splitting the herd into two, separating and—"

Abruptly the Sheikh stood up. Everyone else followed suit as usual. A close member of the Sheikh's family, a nobleman in fine robes lined with gold, had entered. Dr. Gotting beckoned to me to return to my place. The nobleman kissed his kinsman the Sheikh and sat down in the seat that I had vacated.

"That's it for today," murmured my companion.

"What? Do you mean my interview is finished?" I replied.

"Yes, that is his first son and there are a couple of imams, religious leaders from Cairo, waiting to come in. You've had your chance for today. We might as well leave."

We slipped out of the room. I stayed for another seven days taking samples from the oryx and the farm for analysis in England, and attended several more audiences, but I never got another chance to plonk myself down in the vacant chair. I was always beaten to it.

Although I had not been able to deal with any cases of actual disease in the oryx, I was able to suggest measures for tackling the next outbreak and, most important, for getting me the material required for diagnosis. I wrote a long report detailing my ideas for cutting out the spread of disease and improving health generally at the farm, and I wrote scathingly about the horses in the royal stables. Copies were sent to the Sheikh and to various government bodies. Then, loaded with samples of oryx droppings, lucerne, hay, blood, barley, and various other possibly useful substances, I returned to England.

After my first visit to Qatar I kept in contact with Dr. Qayyum and his team and sent out drugs and sample bot-

tles to be ready for the next outbreak of disease in the
oryx. Analysis of the food, blood, and droppings had not
brought up anything abnormal.

It was exactly a year later that the next urgent call
came from Qatar. This time there had not been the same
inexplicable delay in seeking help, but still three days had
elapsed before I was requested to fly out without delay.
Six oryx had died, and although no bodies were available for my inspection, tissue specimens and bacterial
swabs had been taken.

At the farm out in the desert nothing had changed.
The clouds of pigeons still filled the sky above the paddocks, camels and goats wandered at will through the farm,
and the sheep were in an even more desperate state than before. Again, the remaining oryx seemed healthy and in good
condition. I examined the bits of lung and other organs
that Dr. Qayyum and Dr. Iftikhar had taken from the
dead animals. It looked like haemorrhagic septicaemia. I
sent portions by air to England and had others processed
at the local hospital laboratory.

There were many sick sheep on the farm. Each day
there was a pile of new carcasses outside the paddock
gates. I walked among the flocks with my stethoscope
and listened to the chests of sick and dying animals. The
fluid noises and harsh roaring of pneumonia were always
to be found. I asked Dr. Iftikhar again about the innumerable pigeons.

"Why can't we cut down the numbers of those birds?"
I demanded.

"The Sheikh will not do it," he replied. "He says they
are essential for the falcons."

The results came back by telex from the English
laboratory. It was haemorrhagic septicaemia in the oryx,
and the swabs taken from their tissues had grown pure
cultures of Pasteurella bacteria. I was finding the same

germ in all the poor sheep that died at the farm, their lungs studded with angry red areas of pneumonia. At least drugs existed to combat the disease.

"I am going to begin a vaccination programme for the oryx," I told Dr. Iftikhar, "and I'm going to give serum and vaccine to every sheep and goat on the farm."

The Pakistani looked dismayed. "It will be necessary first to request permission from His Excellency the Sheikh," he said. "Without permission, which is difficult to obtain, we cannot inject the oryx; he loves them so much."

"It will have to be done," I insisted. "I'll go to the Majlis to have audience with him tonight."

I then learned that in order to avoid injections the foolhardy practice of mixing broad-spectrum antibiotics with the food for the oryx had been adopted. This sounds like a simple way of administering anti-bacterial drugs to nervous or dangerous wild animals, but in a cud-chewing animal the antibiotics kill most of the harmless bacteria in its stomach which are essential for its special type of digestion. The consequences can be serious and often fatal. I wondered whether any of the deaths at Al Zubarrah had been due more to the therapy than to the complaint.

"And unless we do the sheep and goats as well, there's not much point," I carried on. "Think of the improvement in their value as well."

"But vaccinating sheep!" exclaimed Dr. Iftikhar. "There are so many!"

"We are going to do it, you and me," I replied firmly. He looked miserable.

I went to the evening audience alone and eventually bagged the vacant chair beside the Sheikh. Through the interpreter I explained, "I can help your oryx, Your Excellency, but I need to vaccinate all of them and all the sheep and goats. And to do the oryx I would like to have a strong wooden cattle crush built."

For a few seconds the Sheikh pondered and sipped his tea; then he said a few words to the interpreter.

"The interview is over," he said. "His Excellency says you can have what you want. There will be forty men at the farm tomorrow morning to build whatever structure you require. And you can do all the sheep and goats."

The following day, fortified and refreshed by a pile of watermelons, the forty labourers and I built an elaborate tapering cattle crush against one wall of the oryx paddock. At the end of the crush was a trap designed to hold an individual animal while I vaccinated it. Carpenters cut wood to size, some men dug holes for posts, and others unrolled heavy-gauge wire mesh and nailed it to the posts. By midday we were ready to try it out. We carefully drove the herd of oryx into the wide mouth of the crush. As they were pressed in slowly towards the narrow neck they suddenly panicked. In unison they launched themselves at the sides of the crush. As if it were made of paper the whole contraption fell flat before the charging animals. Ten seconds later not a single piece was left standing.

Unharmed and impassive, the oryx gathered in a distant corner of the paddock and surveyed the scene of our fruitless labours. I would have to use the dart-gun. I loaded every syringe I had with a dose of the vaccine and applied a blob of antibiotic jelly to the needle tips. Although the darts were sterile, as they entered the animals' skins they might take in a particle of soil or dust adhering to the hair, and I was not prepared to run the slightest risk of losing any animals from tetanus.

When all was prepared I sent everyone away so that I could move about the oryx paddock quietly and alone, picking off one animal at a time with the minimum disturbance or fuss. That way I could avoid shooting at moving targets. This was important because in each case I wanted to place a subcutaneous injection precisely over the ribs just behind the shoulder. Any reaction to the vaccine in that place would not interfere with movement and would soon disperse. In order not to inject the vaccine too deep I had selected needles only half an inch long which carried fat little collars to control the depth of penetration. One by one I darted the oryx, who were not disturbed by the relatively quiet gas-powered gun. After delivering its contents each syringe fell out of the animal onto the sand and I retrieved it. It was all over in an hour and a half. Within ten days the oryx would be carrying a good level of protective antibodies in their bloodstreams.

I arranged with Dr. Iftikhar for him to repeat the process in two to four weeks and then set off to see about vaccinating the sheep and goats by hand.

"Surely we can leave the vaccination of these animals to the farm men," said Iftikhar. "I'm sure you don't want to go in with all those hundreds of smelly creatures."

"I want to see every animal properly vaccinated and dosed with anti-serum this afternoon," I replied. "I'll do half and you do the others."

"But the men don't really want to catch the sheep." Iftikhar was looking positively awkward.

"All right, then," I said, "I'll catch them and do them myself."

I went into the sheep paddock with a multidose syringe, grabbed a sheep, vaccinated it, and bundled it out of the gate to the watching group of men and Dr. Iftikhar. I did another and another. Still the men watched. It was going to take a long time at this rate to do all the hundreds of sheep, but I was determined that all susceptible animals were going to be done. Eventually the shame-faced knot of men at the gateway came reluctantly in dribs and drabs into the paddock and began catching animals. Dr. Iftikhar filled his syringe, and before long we were whistling through the flock at a fine old rate.

Before leaving for England I walked round the whole of the farm again. The pox-infested birds were still everywhere, both dead and alive. Out in the small irrigated fields where the lucerne for the oryx was grown I walked down the rows of succulent green plants and noticed many plastic bags, some containing small quantities of white powder, lying on the soil. The bags bore bold skull and crossbones symbols in bright red. The white powder was an insecticide containing the extremely dangerous organo-phosphorus type of chemical. The farm workers had used the stuff and then idly dropped the seemingly empty bags as soon as they had finished with them. In places the white powder was actually caked onto the leaves of the lucerne plants. It worried me. This stuff was fine when properly diluted with water and sprayed, but what if the oryx were fed lucerne contaminated with the concentrated powder?

I pointed out the risk to Dr. Iftikhar and he had words with the labourer in charge of the fields. There was no risk, said the labourer, as they were not going to crop that area for quite a while. He would see that the bags were gathered up and that the powder was washed off the leaves in future.

One month later I received a letter from Dr. Qayyum requesting advice on treating animals poisoned with organo-phosphorus insecticides. Three oryx had eaten lucerne contaminated with the chemical and had developed the typical symptoms of poisoning affecting the nervous system. One of the animals had died by the time he wrote the letter and the other two were gravely ill. Unfortunately the letter took two weeks to reach England, and although I immediately cabled detailed advice, once again I was far too late.

Something else once arrived from Qatar. I went down to breakfast to find a small parcel covered with Qatari stamps waiting on the dining table. Shelagh opened it while I poured the coffee, and out fell a brain! Stuck to the noisome object was a stained piece of notepaper. After hurriedly removing the thing and all its wrappings to my office, I scrubbed my hands in iodine soap and pulled on a pair of plastic gloves. Then I read the letter, which was from Dr. Qayyum. The brain was from a dog with suspected rabies and would I kindly confirm or deny, please!

With all the careful rules and regulations designed to keep the British Isles free from the horrific scourge of rabies, here was a mass of putrefying material possibly loaded with active rabies virus delivered to my breakfast table! I telephoned the Ministry of Agriculture immediately. They seemed puzzled as to the correct thing to do.

"None of the rules fit," said one of the Ministry men to whom I spoke.

"It's not from a British dog so an investigation isn't called for," offered another.

"You haven't asked for its importation so you can't be held responsible for not getting a licence," a third reassured me.

"You can't quarantine a rotting brain," said a fourth, plaintively.

In the end they left it to me to deal with. I was dumbfounded. Nobody in the Ministry seemed to care that I might be about to put Rochdale on the map as the place where rabies entered Britain, possibly never again to be eradicated. I took the brain and all the packing paper, put them in a box filled with carbolic acid, and then incinerated the whole thing. If rabies was indeed in that brain, not a virus particle escaped.

15 The Popsicled Whale

ON CHRISTMAS EVE a few weeks after returning from my first trip to Qatar I was attending a fancy-dress party at Flamingo Park dressed as—what else—a sheikh. A call came through from a friend of mine at Vancouver Aquarium who thought that I might be interested in the news that killer whales had been captured in British Columbia. I immediately put through a call to France, for I knew the new Marineland at Antibes was desperately seeking a killer whale for its grand opening. The director at Antibes jumped at the chance.

"Go out to Canada as soon as you can," he said. "At all costs get us a whale."

I dashed off to change out of the Taylor household's clean bedsheets. Half an hour later, with a bag crammed full of drugs and medical paraphernalia as my only luggage, I set off by car for London Airport. With me was Martin Padley, electronics engineer turned dolphin trainer, an enthusiastic and expert handler of marine mammals.

We arrived in Canada on Christmas Day and then made our way by road and then boat to the isolated bay near Pender Harbour where the whales were. We had been directed to get in touch with Bert Gooldrup, a local fisherman who had apparently directed the whale capture. We had no difficulty locating his house. It was like arriving late at a gold rush. The Gooldrup homestead was surrounded by vehicles of every kind—trucks, jeeps, lowloaders carrying whale slings, and cars with dinghies and outboards on their roofs. I felt empty-handed, for there had been no time for me to arrange for a carrying container or other gear for whale transport to be made or shipped out to Canada.

Indoors, Bert's wife was serving an impromptu Christmas dinner to around fifty men from a dozen zoos and marinelands in the United States. Bert told us that he had been in his bathroom shaving the morning before when he heard some unusual noises like muffled explosions in the bay below his house. He looked out the window. During the night there had been a violent storm and the ocean was murky with stirred-up sand. As his eyes accommodated to the dim light, Bert saw something round and dark riding in the sea about a hundred yards offshore. Then he saw another of the objects, and another, rising and falling gently with the waves. As he watched he saw a foggy plume erupt from the upper surface of one of the objects. Whales! Whales in the bay!

He went down to the shingle beach. There were almost twenty-five of them, black and shining like billiard balls, some big with towering dorsal fins, and others quite small like upturned rubber dinghies. Occasionally they rolled over in the water and their white bellies glistened in the lightening dawn. White bellies! And crisply drawn white curls on their sides and round their eyes! These were killer whales! An audacious idea was gripping him. Here was a group of whales of assorted sizes peacefully lying in the sheltered shallow waters of a small bay, instead of out on the high seas where hunters trying to take them alive had found them to be elusive and formidable adversaries. Bert determined to try to catch some of them.

He went to the phone and rang some fisherman friends, telling them to meet him with their boats and a quantity of gear. An hour or so later a small group of boats loaded with literally miles of salmon netting collected in the bay, well away from the whales to avoid disturbing them. Under Bert's command the fishing boats first blocked off the exit to the sea by running a net across the mouth of the bay. Then, very slowly, they cut the bay in half with a net stretching right across the diameter of the rough circle of water. The whales lay in the half of the bay farther from the sea. The men laid more nets, quartering the bay, and then repeated the process yet again. Gradually the whales were restricted to an ever-decreasing area of open water. They ignored the boats and showed no sign of alarm. As the nets came closer to them they floated gently away from the fragile curtain, drifting ever farther into the trap. Of course these highly intelligent creatures knew that the nets were there. They had excellent vision above and below the water surface, acute hearing, and a sonar echo-location system that is the envy of the world's navies. The sound beams that bounced back to them were loaded with every detail of information about the net's depth, thickness, and design. But what had they to fear from the nets? If they wanted to they could have torpedoed through the thin nylon like bullets through tissue paper. It had needed half-inch stainless-steel mesh to catch killer whales off Seattle when the first of their kind had been taken alive by man.

Eventually, without the slightest resistance, the twenty-two whales were confined in an area as big as Piccadilly Circus. At first Bert had thought that the reason for the whales' remarkable visit into the bay was to shelter from the night's storm, but as he inspected the animals more closely he saw another possible reason. Black and yellow instead of black and white, with a skin so shiny that it reflected the clouds quite plainly, a newly born baby killer whale rose and sank in the swell beside its mother. Perhaps the group had come into the calmer waters of the bay to give the mother better conditions for calving. Bert and his companions now proceeded quietly to split up the whales into small groups of two or three by taking nets among the animals. They took pains to keep the baby with its mother and the big bulls with their attendant harems, but there was no trouble and after a few hours it was done. The nets were reinforced by others dropped outside them. The tops of the nets were nailed to logs and the whole improvised arrangement of what were now whale pens was pulled into shore near a small jetty and anchored into place.

Martin and I went down to the shore and looked down at the whale pens from the end of the jetty. The sea was now still and the logs looked like giant matchsticks laid out on a tablecloth for some gargantuan after-dinner trick. Within the various pens the whales lay calmly, frequently rolling onto their backs, snow-white bellies uppermost, in the relaxed posture so typical of killer whales. As we walked out along the booms they heeled over in the water and a large, dark, red-rimmed eye streaming with syrupy tears cleared the surface to watch us. The faint streams of clicking noises made underwater as they talked to one another through the net dividers could be clearly heard in the evening air. Some of the biggest males were enormous monsters almost thirty feet long. Their dorsal fins were soaring black triangles often over a yard high, flopping over at the top under their own weight. For the first time in my life I saw a baby killer. The youngster bobbed and rolled by the side of his mother, diving under the surface from time to time to suckle the richest milk known to science. He wasn't down at the teat for more than a few seconds; his mother pumped out large quantities of milk at a high rate by contracting powerful muscles in her udder. Baby whales don't have to do much sucking; they just open their gullets and Mum does the rest.

Men with rifles were guarding the whale pens. The year before, lower down the coast, captured whales had been released during the night by persons unknown, possibly jealous fishermen or members of a humane society. This time Bert and his colleagues were taking no chances.

Bert joined us as we inspected the whales, and then he gave us the bad news. It had been agreed that the untransportable big males and the mother and baby should be released. Of the other animals, all except one eighteen-foot-long female had already been bagged by the Americans before we arrived. It would have to be the big female or nothing.

We picked our way across the logs to a pen containing the solitary female. My heart dropped when I saw her. She was enormous, long and lean. Most noticeable about her was her skin, which was covered from tip to tail with peculiar spots. She looked as if she had measles! I had never seen such a skin disease previously. What did it signify? I had no idea. Also, the whale was not eating. Certainly she would not accept any of the fish thrown into her pen. They had tried everything—herring, trout, even salmon—but she had not shown any interest in the offerings.

Now I had to make the big decision. Were we to take this animal? There was an awful lot of money involved, not just in the purchase price but also in the air freight. Two and a half tons of live animal, with sufficient equipment to keep it comfortable, would have to be flown across

the whole of Canada and then the Atlantic. No one had
ever attempted to carry a whale as big as this on such a
long journey. And there were only two of us.

I talked to some of the vets who had come from the
great marinelands of Florida and California. Had they any
views on the spotty whale? Close inspection showed the
spots were actually dimples about half an inch in diameter.
They were pale grey in colour against the normal black
background of the skin. No one had any helpful advice.
They were preoccupied with preparations for their own
purchases, anyway. A decision had to be made immediately. The following day all the whales sold would be
moved off, the rest would be released, and the pens broken
up. The fishermen could not give up any more time.
They needed their nets, for the fish were running.

Martin and I stood alone and looked hard at the whale.
It was impossible to take a blood sample from her in the
water, nor could I make any physical examination. All
we could do was look. "If she's taken out of the water
she must be paid for," said Bert. "With the rest sold we
can't afford to waste any more time on just one." I stared
down at the whale and she stared back at me. Her breathing was strong and normal, the excrement was a healthy
bottle-green colour, the gums were a clear deep pink, and
she produced plenty of sticky tears. All these were good
signs. Only the skin and the great length were obstacles
to my decision.

Finally I decided to take her. I agreed with Bert to
pay one third of her price when we took her from the
water, one third at Vancouver Airport, and the final
third after she had been alive for one month in Europe.

I rang France and gave them the news. They were
pleased but had a problem. Their whale pool had developed a serious crack in the bottom. It would not hold

water and must be completely relined, a job which would take several weeks. They badly wanted the whale, but could I find somewhere in England to hold it for a few weeks?

My head was spinning with problems to be solved. While Martin went off to see what could be done about fixing air transport and getting some sort of whale container built on Christmas Day in the backwoods of Canada, I telephoned England. Eventually I found a pool which could conceivably take an eighteen-foot whale for a few weeks. It was at Cleethorpes Zoo in Lincolnshire, an eight-foot-deep plastic sea-lion pool with filtration and chlorination equipment.

Martin came back after some hours. With the aid of the friend from Vancouver Aquarium he had arranged for a framework of metal tubes to be built in Pender Harbour overnight by a co-operative blacksmith. In the framework we would hang a canvas hammock for the whale. The bottom and sides of the framework would be enclosed in what we hoped was a watertight bag of thick plastic. All this Martin had got under way on Christmas Day! In addition a somewhat dubious official of Lufthansa had said that they were prepared to fly us with our animal from Los Angeles to Manchester, but we would somehow have to get ourselves to Los Angeles. Eventually we found an airline flying an old propeller freighter from Vancouver to Los Angeles. That would have to do. But for everything to go smoothly and to avoid our missing the crucial Los Angeles–Manchester flight, we had to be in Vancouver by early afternoon of the next day. This meant a long road journey, then several hours by ferry, and then more road travel. The ferry company agreed to book space for our lorry on the first boat of the morning. The ferry people were adamant about our being on time; they could not wait. That meant that we had to be the first to take our whale from the water early the next morning.

All the whale transporting teams had lorries and cranes ready for the loading. We arranged to share in the hire of a crane, and hired a lorry and driver from Vancouver which was due to arrive early in the morning. The American teams with their masses of complex equipment and numerous staff thought our two-man expedition and makeshift arrangements rather a joke. They also made it clear that we would have to take our place in line for moving whales from the water. The whole batch of pens was to be towed, with the whales still inside, round to the little dock at Pender Harbour. There the cranes and lorries would line up; the jetty could take only one crane and one lorry at a time. It was impossible to predict how long it would take to load each whale, but as were the last to arrive we would be at the end of the queue.

I pointed out to the Americans that we were going on the longest journey of all and that our plane take-off deadlines had to be met. They were transporting by road and could afford to let us go first. Some of them had purchased three or four whales. Could they not see the point in letting us get away first on the following morning with our single animal, the biggest to be taken? No, they couldn't. It was just our hard luck.

Martin and I retired to consider. It hardly seemed worthwhile trying; we were bound to miss the ferry and hence the other connections. Nonetheless, we decided to continue making our preparations. Perhaps something would turn up.

We worked through the late evening and night getting things in order for the morning. Meanwhile the American teams, their gear completely shipshape and ready, went out to celebrate Christmas some miles away at an inn. They must have enjoyed themselves, for it was three o'clock in the morning when they returned and went to bed to sleep it off. Martin and I instantly realized that this was our chance. The revellers would no doubt sleep well and deeply. Surely they would not be rising briskly at daybreak. We, however, would be up early. We arranged to begin the operation at the crack of dawn.

At the first lightening of the sky we rose and quietly left the cabin near the Gooldrups' house where we had been quartered along with most of the others. Our lorry had arrived and with it the hastily assembled whale container. We drove everything down to Pender Harbour and before anyone was about backed our lorry into position on the jetty. Martin found the crane driver and persuaded him to get his machine into place next to the lorry. We were ready. When the Americans and the whale pens arrived they would find us *in situ* on the jetty.

Some time later the boats towing the floating pens appeared at the mouth of the harbour. The whales maintained their positions in the centres of their pens and slowly cruised along with the whole contraption. It was weird how compliantly these powerful creatures went along with their captors' machinations. They might easily have rammed their way through the salmon netting even though it had been reinforced; instead, seemingly still unalarmed, they were content with not allowing themselves to come in contact with the nets around them.

Last came the Americans. They protested furiously, but we were in possession of the jetty, and the ignition keys of lorry and crane were in my pocket.

The whale pens filled the little harbour. There were sixteen whales in all; the others had been released but followed events at a distance, leaping completely out of the water as if to obtain a better view of what was going on. The fishermen manoeuvred the pen containing our whale next to the jetty end. They slipped more nets into the pen and gradually brought them up beneath the animal; two or three nets alone would not have been sufficient to stand the strain soon to be put upon them.

The crane lowered a cable which was attached to the nets, and then with surprisingly little fuss the lift began. As the whale felt the netting touch her belly she wriggled and beat her massive tail on the water surface, drenching the men in the surrounding small boats. Up she came; then she was clear of the water and the nets took her full weight. But we were going to have difficulties transferring her from the net to the hammock. I was afraid of cutting her delicate skin if we dragged the net out from under her once she was in position, so I decided to put her back into the water and put the hammock in after her.

The nets were lowered until there was about a foot of clear water beneath the whale, and then Martin, already dressed in his rubber wet suit, jumped in and began to fit the hammock around her. It had been made to size for her according to our estimations of her length and girth. There were holes for her flippers, eyes, and vent. Bit by bit Martin teased the big sheet of canvas into place. Like a mammoth meatball sieved out of the pot, she hung, resting comfortably and glaring at us through the eye holes. Her belly bulged out of the vent hole.

The crane driver took the great submarine shape, streaming sea water, high above the water, up to the jetty, and then over to where I was standing by the lorry, holding her above my head as I took a blood sample from the underside of her tail flukes. Then the loading continued. The whale in her hammock was placed into the framework, and we took the lorry off the jetty so that the Americans could get on with fishing out their whales.

The catch had been an unexpected bonanza for the little ice-making plant in Pender Harbour. Normally active only during the summer, the plant had been at full stretch over Christmas churning out ice in crushed form for the needs of the whale buyers. In air, a poorer heat conductor than water, whales have difficulty getting rid of their waste heat and could literally boil to death by developing an excessive temperature rise in their internal organs. To avoid this they are kept cool by the application of ice and water during transport.

We had purchased 500 pounds of ice. After the whale had been adjusted in the hammock, I covered her with wet cotton sheets and then packed crushed ice around her. Reserve ice was carried in big plastic trash bins. We installed a recirculating water spray system over the whale by means of a bilge pump, twelve-volt battery, and lengths of plastic pipe with holes punched in the wall. This device kept a flow of chilly water constantly squirting over her back. The water then ran down the sides and dripped into the bottom of the plastic-surrounded container, where it was sucked up again by the bilge pump.

As we hurried to make things as pleasant as possible for our whale's long journey, we heard the sounds of commotion coming from the jetty. The whales were at last beginning to lose their cool. The second whale to be loaded was causing trouble. It was charging the net and upsetting the fishing boats. We told the driver to set off for the ferry. We had no wish to endure the wrath of the American teams if things went badly from now on. Later we learned that the animal did in fact escape and make off to sea with the big bulls and the mother and baby.

Off we rattled on the back of the lorry. It was intensely cold, particularly once we were moving. Martin and I busied ourselves protecting the most sensitive areas of the whale's skin from damage and drying. We plastered Vaseline round the "armpits" and blowhole, covered the eyes with soothing, greasy, antibiotic cream, and packed cotton wool and foam plastic between the canvas edges and the bulging stomach. The plan was to stop at a hospital when we neared civilization and have a fast blood analysis begun on the sample I had taken. We could then drive on, telephoning for results from the airport, before paying the second instalment on the price.

But it was not to be. Possibly because the driver had zealously tried to give the whale a gentle ride through the wooded hills on the way to the ferry and had kept his foot on the brakes down every long incline and round each hairpin bend, the brakes suddenly failed. The rest of the journey was rather hairy. The driver used his gears as brakes, but there was no time to stop at the hospital. We made the ferry in time and, with a display of masterly though unorthodox driving, eventually reached the airport in Vancouver.

The plane was a nose loader, and with the aid of special lifting devices our cargo was soon packed safely on board. Because of the whale's heat production, much of the ice originally packed round her had melted and the container was now awash with dozens of gallons of icy water. Before take-off I gave the animal several injections—antistress compounds, anti-pneumonia shots, and a massive dose of vitamin B_1 six thousand times stronger than a normal adult human dose—and asked the flight engineer to adjust the cargo hold air temperature at 0 degrees centigrade. It would be best for the whale but miserable for us.

The plane taxied down the runway and took off, lifting its nose up into a blue sky. The climbing angle made the water and mushy ice in the whale container swill back, and it came pouring over the end of the plastic shrouding.

Scrambling up the sloping floor of the still-climbing air-craft, Martin and I struggled to hold the plastic up and keep the water in, but it was impossible. Water spilled over us and rushed down towards the rear of the aircraft.

The plane soon levelled out and the water settled down again. We added more ice to the container and continually checked to see that every portion of the whale's anatomy was being kept wet. Then I noticed that the water glisten-ing on the whale's skin was actually beginning to freeze; ice crystals were sticking to the skin cells. The temperature of the compartment had dropped too low, which could mean serious frost damage to the whole of the skin surface above water level. Martin went forward to see the engineer, and a few minutes later I was relieved to see the ice crystals on the skin begin to melt.

The journey to Los Angeles was not very long, and the Lufthansa 707 for the next stage of our flight was ready upon our arrival, as was a further supply of ice courtesy of friends at Los Angeles Marineland of the Pacific. Boeing 707 aircraft are not nose loaders; the cargo door is on the side, and when we attempted to transfer our living bundle of freight I had a horrible shock. The whale framework was too big for the door! No matter how the expert load-ers tried, even unbolting portions of the fuselage at the door edges, the thing would not go in. My nightmare of being stranded with a whale seemed likely to be fulfilled. There was only one thing to be done. We would have to cut off one third of the rigid framework supporting the whale in her hammock, leaving the tail end of the animal flopping about inside the outer plastic bag. Then, once loaded, we would somehow have to rope the bag up to the ceiling of the aircraft.

Cutting the tubes of the framework and adjusting the supports meant two hours of work with acetylene torches and metal saws. The noise was appalling. I felt sorry for the poor whale: what could she have been thinking? Nevertheless she lay calmly throughout, breathing easily and squeaking from time to time in the querulous pig-like manner of her kind. I found that she appreciated being squeaked back at and would answer squeaks made by me with noises of similar type and duration.

Eventually we completed the modifications. Now the container looked like a jungle gym that had been dynamited. Bits of rope and metal were jumbled together, and the plastic outer shell flopped and bulged and trailed all over the place. Loading of the 707 went ahead smoothly now. The next thing was a delay due to heavy air traffic; we eventually set off three hours late.

The journey seemed interminable, first back up into Canada to Montreal, where we loaded more freight and I bought extra supplies of ice, and then on through the night over the Atlantic towards Britain. Both Martin and I were exhausted. We took turns snatching a few minutes' sleep curled up on the uncomfortable metal floor of the jet freighter. Every few hours I gave the whale more injections, but tranquillizers weren't necessary; she seemed as settled as a seasoned globe-trotter.

Then problems started again. The navigator came back to give us some news. First, we would not be landing at Manchester but at London. However, he would radio ahead when within range to inform our friends in England of the change in plans, so that they could move the waiting lorry and equipment from Manchester to London. An hour later the navigator came back again. Because of the delay in starting, our ETA in London would be early in the morning, long before the authorities would permit landing at Heathrow, because of noise restrictions on night flying. So the aircraft would go on to Frankfurt, unload the whale so that other cargo could be handled, reload the whale, and then, when Heathrow was open, fly on to London. This was too much. I went forward.

"Captain, this is going to make matters critical for the animal," I said. "I don't like the look of her condition. Can't you make a special landing at London?"

"Only in an emergency," he replied.

I thought of my poor, patient whale and the extra hours that would be added to the already extended journey. A white or even greyish lie seemed justified. "I don't think she'll make Frankfurt. Even London will be a close call. The respiration isn't what it should be and it looks like broncho-pneumonia."

The captain was sympathetic and very concerned, but he was certain that London would not give permission to land.

"Will Lufthansa want to be responsible for the carcass if we land and she's dead?" I asked. I regretted having to press him in this way, but I had no alternative.

The captain shrugged. He looked worried. "I'll do my best with Heathrow but . . ."

I returned to the whale. We did not have much ice left now, and I hoped that the people meeting us would have brought enough for the long road journey to Cleethorpes. Martin was having trouble keeping the water circulating. At this stage in a shipment the pump and the holes in the plastic tubing become increasingly clogged with particles of excrement from the whale. Much of our time was spent poking the holes free with bits of wire. Every half hour we had to strip down the bilge pump and clean it. We were wet and exhausted, covered with grease, and stinking of whale faeces.

As we neared London the navigator came to us smiling. London had given special permission to land. Saved again! Soon we would be on the ground and could go to bed for a few hours while the team meeting us took over responsibility for unloading the whale and taking her by road to the final destination. As we landed at Heathrow and taxied to a halt, Martin and I slapped one another's backs. We had done it! The end was in sight. Only one small lap to go.

We waited expectantly as the cargo door slid upwards and the customs officer boarded. We looked out onto the tarmac. Where were the familiar faces? Where was the van? Not a soul was in sight. Perhaps our people were in the customs shed and would meet us there or were waiting for permission to come on to the airfield. The cargo handlers arrived and we asked them. No, they didn't know of anybody waiting for us. Tired as I was, I could have hopped about in a white-hot rage. What had happened?

A little while later a car dashed onto the airfield and came over to where we were standing watching the whale container being carefully slid out of the hold of the 707. In the car was the director of the Antibes Marineland.

"Roland, where the devil is everybody?" I asked, as he jumped out. "Where is the lorry?"

He grimaced. "It's up in Manchester, or at least it was. We got the message about the change of destination too late to stop the driver. He was already on his way to Manchester airport. Anyway, we're going to hire another one, and some keepers from Cleethorpes will be here shortly by car to give you a hand."

We waited while the lorry was obtained. It was another open vehicle. At least that would help to keep the whale's temperature down, for we were running short of ice and our fresh supplies were in Manchester. As sufficient ice was not to be found at that hour in Heathrow, we decided to set off to the north with the little we had and see how we went on. The whale was loaded once more and after Customs had inspected her, looked inside the crate, I suppose for smuggled goods, counted her, scratched their heads over classifying her in their tariff books, and generally delayed us still more, we drove towards the M.1 freeway.

It was a cold night, and soon heavy rain began to fall. It was highly unpleasant tending the whale on the back of an open lorry under these conditions, but it suited the whale fine. I had a thermometer with which I frequently checked the temperature of the water in the bottom of the container. Some mushy ice still floated in it and the reading was 0 degrees centigrade, but I was down to my last ten pounds of crushed ice. We reached the motorway and turned north. Still it rained, and the men clinging to the whale container were bitterly cold and wet.

As we approached Watford Gap I could see that the whale was beginning to steam a little in the torchlight beam. Hot areas such as her forehead and flippers were drying out quicker than before. There were small cracks appearing round the blowhole. I tested the water again. The temperature was 10 degrees centigrade. I could find no floating ice in the dim light, and my ice reserves were spent. We had at least another hundred miles to go, but where could one obtain a sufficient quantity of ice at three o'clock in the morning on a motorway?

We were almost at a service station. I told the driver to pull in there and we would see if they had any ice. The motorway restaurant manager was very apologetic but they had none. Then I had an idea. Had they got any popsicles?

"How many would you need?" said the manager. "We've cases of them in the deep-freeze."

"About a thousand," I replied, "but the flavours don't matter."

The manager gulped, said nothing, and disappeared. Five minutes later and £50 lighter we were loading boxes of orange, strawberry, and lime popsicles onto the lorry. "We've just about enough of these things to keep the temperature down until we reach Cleethorpes," I told the men, "so we'll drive straight through without any stops for coffee." And so we rolled on through the night with the whale, who had by then been named Calypso by Roland, wallowing in a multicoloured sludge of melting ice and popsicle sticks.

Calypso arrived safely at Cleethorpes and with the aid of a crane was released into the pool prepared for her. Martin and I stood grinning as she swam gracefully out of the hammock and began to cruise slowly round. Now I would have a chance to thoroughly examine her and get her in good shape before she made her final trip to Antibes and the sunny skies of the Côte d'Azur.

Cleethorpes is a bleak place in winter. The cold wet wind from the North Sea harries the small zoo situated by the water's edge as it streams inland. The reserve sea-lion pool at the zoo had been filled with fresh sea water ready for Calypso's arrival. It was icy cold, ideal for killer whales but punishing for those of us who had to treat the animal and begin the process of acclimatizing her. Unlike Cuddles, the first killer whale to arrive in England, Calypso showed not the slightest interest in feeding when released into the Cleethorpes pool. Round and round she swam, sometimes turning her head slightly to watch a thrown-in herring or mackerel drop through the water but never once opening her mouth.

Now my health programme for Calypso began in earnest. I had several worries about her. My blood samples showed her to be anaemic, and there was the peculiar skin disease. But worst of all was the lack of appetite. Whales

can go for long periods without feeding. They store energy
in a highly efficient manner in their layers of blubber, a sort
of concentrated fatty tissue. In time of starvation these reserves are drawn upon and the blubber layer slowly becomes thinner. The thinner the blubber the less insulation
the animal has against the cold surrounding water, and a
vicious circle of accelerating heat and energy loss may set
in. There was also the problem of dehydration. Whales and
dolphins can safely drink sea water, discharging the excessive amount of salt, which would kill human beings,
through specially adapted kidneys and bowels. They also
get water by chemical reaction as a by-product when their
food intake is burnt and processed by the body. No food
meant no water-producing processes.

I had to get her eating. For the first two weeks we
tried tempting Calypso with all kinds of fish: herring, whit-
ing, even whole salmon. We released live fish into the pool.
Still no sign of interest. Each day the pool was drained so
that I could examine Calypso as she lay on the bottom. I
gave her injections of vitamins and other drugs through a
hypodermic needle twelve inches long and thick as a knitting needle. We put a sea-lion in with her to see if that
would stimulate an interest in eating. The only result was
that the sea-lion chased her round the pool, nipping her tail
and sometimes hitching rides on the broad black back.
At last I could wait no longer. Weight loss was beginning to show distinctly. I would have to begin force-
feeding.

So began a laborious programme of intensive care.
Now the pool had to be drained twice a day and a long plastic tube passed down into the whale's stomach. After much
effort we found that the way to make the whale open her
mouth was to squirt water between her tightly clenched
jaws from a hosepipe. She didn't seem to like the cold jet

on her palate and would fleetingly open her mouth. Then, in a flash, we pushed in a big teak-wood gag. It was not easy. Calypso would wave her head about in annoyance, cracking our legs with the ends of the wooden billet. Four men had to hold onto the gag desperately in order to keep it from being dislodged. Through a hole in the centre of the gag the tube was passed into the stomach. A stirrup pump was attached and then, slowly, to avoid regurgitation, a large binful of nourishing liquid was pumped down into the whale. The liquid I used was a soup of invalid food, honey, glucose, liquid protein, vitamins, and Guinness. After the first week of force-feeding I added whole raw herring which had been homogenized in an electric blender.

Still Calypso showed no sign of voluntary eating. The weather worsened, with snow or sleet falling daily, accompanied by bitter winds. Each day I checked for the first symptoms of dehydration by taking blood and looking for the telltale signs of water shortage. It didn't happen, and gradually the anaemia improved under injection treatment.

At the beginning of the third week I decided to commence force-feeding of whole fish. This entailed putting my arm down Calypso's throat. I put it through the hole in the gag, and it was awkward, but the gag did keep one's arm intact. Martin and I began by using herring but changed quickly to the firmer mackerel. We made progress. Bit by bit Calypso learned to swallow the fish more and more easily. Eventually they had only to be placed on the tongue. We changed to coalfish. Calypso began to accept the gag and would even put out her tongue slightly to receive the food. Then came the great day. Before the regular first draining of the day, Martin tried the whale with a coalfish dropped into the water. She took it, sucking it into her mouth in a swirl of water. We celebrated with champagne. ˙m now on treatment could be easily continued by putting drugs and vitamins in the fish and Martin could begin training her by reward to do a few tricks, even though the pool was shallow.

Slowly the skin dimples on Calypso faded. Microscopic examination of portions of the affected skin had not given us the answer as to the nature of the complaint so our treatment had to be speculative. Now, six years later, we think it was indeed measles, the same virus condition that attacks children.

It was three months before Calypso was able to go on the next stage of her journey to France. A special charter plane took her to Nice. She was ceremoniously escorted to her new home by the fire chief and his men, who in France are responsible for everything having to do with water—including whales, it seems. In a thunderstorm probably as bad as the one which had led to her being captured in the first place, Calypso was released into a gigantic deep pool of water. Martin and I swam alongside her after she had been freed from the hammock. After nuzzling us gently with her snub black nose, she swung round and, seeing the expanse of blue water available to her, zoomed off joyously in a flat-out, upside down lap of honour.

Envoi

IT HAS BEEN MY PRIVILEGE to know and to treat many animals like Calypso, Mimi the sea-lion, and Suzy the gorilla, and to watch them return to strength and health. Sometimes, no matter what I have done for a patient, I have failed, but such moments of despair have been amply made up for by the good times, by the creatures from tortoise to elephant that I have been able to help. The real reward is the strengthening pulse of a gorilla that was lying critically ill from pneumonia or the alligator whose eye, once a blind mass of bloody tumour, now watches you malignantly through a clear and limpid cornea. Every day I learn something new in the vast world of exotic animals. Every day I learn something more and find out how little I know about the rich variety of animal species and their numberless diseases.

There is much to be done, many problems to be solved. What is the secret of the deadly liver disease of cheetahs and the hepatitis of dolphins? Why do so few exotic species breed well in captivity? What is the real nature of so many of the unstudied diseases of reptiles and amphibians?

I do not know the answers to these and many other questions, and perhaps I never will, but the most exciting thing in life is trying to find out.